Challenges and Innovations
in U.S. Health Care

Also of Interest

*Health for the Whole Person: The Complete Guide to Holistic Medicine, edited by Arthur C. Hastings, James Fadiman, and James S. Gordon

*Interpersonal Behavior and Health Care, Michael A. Counte and Luther P. Christman

*Systems of Health Care, Douglas R. Mackintosh

*Behavioral Intervention in Health Care, Laura B. Gordon

*Health Care Delivery Systems, J. C. Salloway

*Hospital Organization and Health Care Delivery, Luther P. Christman and Michael A. Counte

*The Dynamics of Aging: Original Essays on the Processes and Experiences of Growing Old, Forrest J. Berghorn, Donna E. Schafer, and Associates

Assuring Quality Ambulatory Health Care: The Martin Luther King Jr. Health Center, edited by Donald Angehr Smith and Gitanjali Mukerjee

*Politics, Science, and Cancer: The Laetrile Phenomenon, edited by Gerald E. Markle and James C. Petersen

Psychosocial Aspects of Drug Treatment for Hyperactivity, edited by Kenneth D. Gadow and Jan Loney

Health Goals and Health Indicators: Policy, Planning, and Evaluation, edited by Jack Elinson, Anne Mooney, and Athilia E. Siegmann

Assessing the Contributions of the Social Sciences to Health, edited by M. Harvey Brenner, Anne Mooney, and Thomas J. Nagy

Impacts of Program Evaluation on Mental Health Care, edited by Emil J. Posavac

The Myths of Deinstitutionalization: Policies for the Mentally Disabled, edited by Joseph Halpern, Karen L. Sackett, Paul R. Binner, and Cynthia B. Mohr

*Available in hardcover and paperback.

Westview Special Studies in Health Care and Medical Science

Challenges and Innovations in
U.S. Health Care
edited by Allen W. Imershein

Increased concern in the 1960s about the quality and availability of health care in the United States prompted a variety of attempts to develop new policies and to modify the existing health care system. The authors of this book review some of those attempts and provide critical commentary on a broad range of new and continuing problems. Their succinct review of many vital aspects of the current health care system clearly demonstrates the successes and failures of health care policy and its impact on the overall system.

The authors discuss consumer involvement in the health care system, the development of neighborhood health clinics, health maintenance organizations and health systems agencies, veterans' medical care, chiropractic, the use of non-physicians in care, changing ideologies among physicians, and the impact of health education. A variety of analytical perspectives are used to evaluate the many issues raised, ranging from a highly critical Marxist commentary on fundamental flaws in the U.S. health system to a pluralist analysis of how the current system might be made to work better.

Dr. Allen W. Imershein is associate professor of sociology at Florida State University. He was a visiting scholar in the Department of Health Administration at the University of North Carolina at Chapel Hill during 1980-81 and is currently engaged in research on organizational change and social reform in human services. His previous publications include Power, Paradigms, and Community Research: Some Patterns Among Recent Studies (edited with Roland J. Liebert) and New Organizational Avenues for Health Education (with Jerry W. Davis).

Challenges and Innovations in U.S. Health Care

edited by Allen W. Imershein

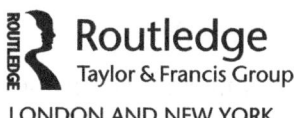

Routledge
Taylor & Francis Group
LONDON AND NEW YORK

Westview Special Studies in Health Care and Medical Science

First published 1981 by Westview Press

Published 2018 by Routledge
52 Vanderbilt Avenue, New York, NY 10017
2 Park Square, Milton Park, Abingdon, Oxon OX14 4RN

Routledge is an imprint of the Taylor & Francis Group, an informa business

Library of Congress Catalog Card Number: 81-52517
ISBN: 978-0-865-31322-4

ISBN 13: 978-0-367-01902-0 (hbk)
ISBN 13: 978-0-367-16889-6 (pbk)

Contents

Tables

Challenges and Innovations
in U.S. Health Care

1
American Health Care: Paradigm Structures and the Parameters of Change

Allen W. Imershein   Florida State University

Recent commentary on the health care scene in the United States has moved increasingly toward explanations of why little or no change has occurred, despite many declarations of crisis." From Alford's (1975) elitist analysis in Health Care Politics to Navarro's (1976) Marxist analysis in Medicine Under Capitalism, critics in and out of the social sciences have tried to make sense of the array of current problems and the apparent lack of response to them. These analyses are in striking contrast to earlier commentaries (e.g., Schwartz, 1971; Garfield, 1970; Anderson, 1972; Citizens Board, 1972) that, although highly critical of then current health care arrangements, foresaw the potential for change within the system and often made recommendations for potential solutions. These earlier analyses might have been characterized by an unwarranted optimism regarding the potential for change, but recent analyses have more than counter-balanced that orientation with an overwhelming skepticism regarding the likelihood of any significant change, short of a major societal restructuring. From the elitist perspective, Alford sees our health care system as rooted in the distribution of power and control in the United States; from a Marxist perspective, Navarro sees the fundamental economic structure of the society as the basis for the current health care system. Thus both believe that no significant change should have been, nor can be, expected.

Despite such criticisms, there have been increasing attempts made in the public arena to change the delivery of health care. Government involvement in financing (actual and proposed), the development of health maintenance organizations (again often under government sponsorship), the establishment of health systems agencies as regulatory organizations, the training of physician extenders and other new allied paraprofessionals, the emergence of family practice as a specialty, and the renewed interest in health education are all examples of the immense energy apparently directed toward answering perceived health care needs. For a field in which current critics tell us there is little potential for significant change, there appears to be a lot going on. The chapters[1] in this book report some of those "goings on." What is particularly notable about them is that the analytical perspectives and value commitments of the authors are as widely varied as the studies themselves, and probably reflect the range of perspectives in the larger health care arena. Some of the studies have no particular theoretical commitments, while at least two (Lasker and MacDougall) identify themselves in some fashion with a Marxist perspective, and one (Bodenheimer and Dixon) is avowedly Marxist. Also, some of the analyses are based on the framework of "established" assumptions currently espoused by major segments of the health care system, even when the analyses criticize implementation within that framework; others challenge even the most basic assumptions. The conclusions drawn from such different approaches are, needless to say, vastly different. The contents of this volume reflect both the range of issues and the range of approaches that characterize the ongoing changes and conflicts in the health care arena. We have not attempted to provide any definitive answers on the significance of current changes or on definitive methods for examining the questions, which may or may not actually be answerable. Rather, we have tried to provide some examples of how different people have gone about accomplishing that task.

In this introductory chapter, I will briefly review the major points and perspectives addressed in the following chapters, and then try to provide a general framework one might use for addressing the questions of change and significance.

RECENT STUDIES OF INNOVATION AND CHANGE

The first several chapters focus on specific attempts at change or innovation. Most of these attempts were made in response to a range of perceived problems in the health care system. The litany is a familiar one: maldistribution of physicians both geographically and across specialities, inaccessibility of care, excess cost to consumers, lack of prevention, spiralling costs, lack of coordination and integration of services (see, for example, Heal Yourself, 1973; or Ehrenreich and Ehrenreich, 1970). Together these elements constitute the major characteristics cited as evidence of a health

---

[1]Most of these were first presented as papers in the Health, Health Policy, and Health Services Division of the Society for the Study of Social Problems, August, 1979.

care crisis, and they have provided either the instiga-
tion or the legitimation for a great variety of reform
attempts.

In Chapter 2, Bebe Lavin looks at the need for and
potential of non-physician primary care assistance. The
lack of available physicians, especially for primary
care; the possibility of using physicians' time more
efficiently by allocating non-essential tasks to less
highly trained personnel; and the desire to include less
technical, more wholistic elements in the care process,
have all contributed to growing pressure for non-physician
professionals. Given that primary-care visits are estimated to constitute 60 percent of all physician visits
and that some estimate that 60 to 80 percent of requests
at these visits could be handled by someone other than a
physicians, the potential for the use of less highly
trained personnel, such as physician assistants or family
nurse practitioners, seems great indeed. However, Lavin
finds significant tension underlying such practices and
limiting their potential: the question of public acceptance. Those who are most educated and most knowledgable
about their own health (the middle and upper classes) are
more willing to accept non-physician care; but given the
existing problems of physician distribution, they are
also the least likely to receive such alternative care.
Instead, rural dwellers and the urban poor, who are on
the whole less educated and less willing to forego the
authority and expertise attributed to a physician, are
most likely to be exposed to non-physician care because
of the local scarcity of physicians. Lavin examines the
problems encountered here and considers the conditions
that would make public acceptance more likely.

Health maintenance organizations (HMO's) have been in
existence for many years, but only recently has the
federal government become involved in encouraging their
development. HMOs are seen as a method of organizing
care in order to reduce costs, increase consumer accountability, and improve the quality of care, especially by
emphasizing preventive rather than crisis care. In
Chapter 3, Judith Barr and Marcia Steinberg examine the
implementation of HMOs with particular emphasis on the
impact it has had on physician autonomy. Autonomy is a
central issue because it is defined (following Freidson,
1970) as the core characteristic essential to the
physician's role as an independent professional. When a
new organizational program involving bureaucratization
and government intervention is seen as challenging traditional physician roles and authority, the implications
of that program approach are taken very seriously by
the medical profession (cf. the long history of AMA opposition to HMO type structures). Barr and Steinberg argue
that, in fact, little threat is posed to physician autonomy by HMOs because physicians for the most part are

able to control both the process and the results of HMO implementation. Professional norms may be challenged, but their authority appears to be maintained.

In Chapter 4, Bonnie Edington examines the confusion generated by a legislative mandate that demanded the conflicting goals of achieving containment, quality improvement, and greater accessibility at the same time. Planning and coordination emerged as a high priority in the 1960s, and as a result the Comprehensive Health Planning Agencies came into being. These agencies were replaced in the mid-1970s by Health Systems Agencies (HSAs) under the National Health Planning Act of 1974. HSAs were supposedly designed to plan and coordinate health services in designated areas throughout the country. But here as elsewhere contradictions abound, and sometimes prevail. Attempts to improve service while also reducing costs have often resulted in simple stagnation. A major upshot of the inability to do both has been a tendency to blame the victim for "overusing" health care services (thus raising costs), for eating improperly and following "unhealthy" lifestyles, and so on. Edington provides an overview of the development of the HSAs, analyzes the contradictions, and considers the results of the process.

One of the more widely hailed health care innovations of the 1960s was the development of neighborhood health centers (NHCs). As part of the "Great Society" program, NHCs were seen as a means to make low-cost health care more available to low income groups, particularly in badly underserved and explosive inner-city neighborhoods. They were to be organized in a fashion that would be responsive to neighborhood needs, that would encourage citizen participation, and that would provide local employment. To say that Tom Bodenheimer and Marlene Dixon came to negative conclusions about the reality of these NHCs is to state the case mildly. The authors of the first three chapters have taken no explicit theoretical position, but Bedenheimer ad Dixon provide a clearly Marxist critique that is both vehement and biting. Using case analysis, they argue that NHCs have failed to be responsive and to provide needed care, and worse, they have served as vehicles for government exploitation of the poor and as tools for domestic counterinsurgency. In their opinion, since the health care system is presently controlled by dominant political and economic interests, we should not have expected otherwise.

In Chapter 6, Judith Lasker tackles the Veterans Administration. Just as the National HMO Act was built upon earlier models of HMO activity, so other systems and organizations serve as models for potential national health care financing or health care services. The Veterans Administration is our main existing government-financed, federally run system within the free "enterprise" health environment. Lasker examines the dynamics of VA functioning and evaluates its potential as a model for a national health service. Those who favor a national health service have often cited the VA as an example of successful government financing and management in the health care field, but Lasker sees problems in using the VA as a model. The VA has been subject to the influence, if not the control, of dominant political, economic, military, and medical interests and therefore has not necessarily been organized to best serve the interests and needs of the veterans for whom it supposedly exists. Lasker suggests that a national service modeled in similar fashion would suffer from similar conflicts in management and wind up failing to serve the public it was intended for.

With a growing elderly population we have become increasingly concerned about care for the elderly and for dying patients. Patient-physician communication and interaction have also become central concerns to many of us. In Chapter 7, John MacDougall examines changes in physician ideologies regarding interaction and communication with dying patients as a means to explain, and as an indicator of, general changes in patterns of physician behavior. In particular, MacDougall finds evidence that current physician ideologies favor more openness toward dying patients and greater coordination with professional teams, reflecting structural changes in the organization of care. Physicians are now less independent, and must rely on technological equipment and bureaucratic settings that are in turn dependent upon corporate and government funding. Changing physician ideologies can thus be linked to underlying challenges to the traditional character of medical practice and are indicative of the corporatization of medicine.

If medicine has been challenged from within, it has also been challenged from without. In a follow-up of his now classic article, Walter Wardwell examines the development and status of one of medicine's principal outside challengers: chiropractic. While at one time it was relegated to the status of a marginal health profession, as Wardwell earlier had characterized it, chiropractic has evolved to the status of a chief rival of orthodox medicine. Evidence of this success lies in the accreditation of its colleges, its being granted reimbursement status under medicare, and the achievement of licensing authority in all states. Both the challenging, confrontive tactics of chiropractic and its overt and vocal rejection by orthodox medicine have subsided. The more general acceptance and use of chiropractic may indicate either a movement of chiropractic toward orthodox medicine (for which there is little evidence) or a willingness of the public to seek beyond orthodox medicine (which is more likely the case). As Wardwell notes, the triumph of chiropractic provides fascinating commentary on the status of orthodox medicine.

In Chapter 9, Ann Ford and Scott Ford take a look at

who's practicing what they preach when it comes to healthy life-styles. Potentially preventable (and not easily curable) diseases are now the major causes of morbidity and mortality in this country, and we are also concerned with alleged over-use of health care facilities and the need to reduce or at least contain the costs of health care. Therefore there has been growing interest in disease prevention, healthy life-styles, and health education. While the general public may acknowledge these concerns, Ford and Ford found that healthy life-style practices may be observed more in the telling than in the doing. Those who know what healthful practices are do not always engage in them. Moreover, a consistent correlation of high levels of tension with unhealthy life-style habits (e.g., smoking and snacking), and an inverse relation between tension and healthful practices (e.g., exercise and seat belt use) suggests that there may be external factors that determine whether an individual will choose a healthy life-style. Health education may be proposed as a useful tool for improving our national health, but modification of other, more systemic factors may be necessary before any significant change can occur.

In Chapter 10, Al Imershein and Gina Miller consider two aspects of the movement for increased consumer involvement in health care that appear to be potentially challenging to current arrangements. Imershein and Miller examine the participation of consumers in the organization of health care and look at the self-care movement. The addition of health care consumers to decision-making bodies was initially hailed as a breakthrough that would increase the responsiveness of health care organizations to consumer needs, but the ineffectiveness of such bodies or their continued dominance by health care providers has blocked any real change. However, the self-care movement, which focuses on practices essentially independent of traditional health care, may have long-term viability and potential for change, if it does not evoke active opposition or provoke attempts at cooptation by the medical establishment.

Obviously the range of issues considered in this volume is only representative of the full range of issues in health care today. But the character of those changes and the major perspectives on the issues are well represented by this collection of papers. I would now like to look at how some of these issues relate to the positive and negative general critiques of the overall health care arena I noted at the outset.

PARADIGM STRUCTURES IN AMERICAN HEALTH CARE

Elsewhere (Imershein, 1977a, 1977b) I have argued the utility of conceptualizing American health care as an organizational paradigm, following Kuhn's (1970) analysis of scientific paradigms. That framework is useful here, I believe, for examining both the limited potential for significant change and the actual appearance of a wide array of more limited changes. First, American medical practice can best be understood as a paradigm community, with physicians, medical educators, and hospital administrators as the primary community members and with the general public acting in response to this community. Second, as a paradigm community, the medical establishment's major activities are ordered by virtue of widely shared, taken-for-granted models of practice. Third, these dominant models are in turn intrinsically linked to certain assumptions about the nature of health, illness, and medicine and about how physicians and health care (or more narrowly, medical care) should be related to the larger society. Finally, given the dominance of this paradigm community within the larger society, these practices and assumptions are established as well by custom, by rule of law, by influence over the ongoing political process, and by some control of economic resources relevant to the area of practice.

Change in this paradigm community can occur in two different ways. First, there are the changes that occur as the result of the "natural" development of the paradigm; for example, the extension of existing patterns of practice to relatively new areas or the development of new modes of practice based upon and consistent with existing arrangements (see Kuhn, 1970: Ch. 3, for a discussion of scientific paradigm development). Second, major changes - those fundamentally altering existing practices - only occur through revolution; that is, through rejection of the dominant paradigm and acceptance of a new one. Such change only comes after an extended period of crises during which numerous unresolvable problems (Khun: anomalies) arise. These problems are unresolvable by the community members but nonetheless demand resolution. Alternative models of practice considered at this point may form the basis for a new paradigm. (For more detail on this process, please see Imershein, 1977a, 1977b; Kuhn, 1970).

Given this framework, opportunities for significant change within the health arena can be seen as severely limited. It may be extremely difficult to modify the political and economic linkages established between the paradigm community and the larger society (the focus for elitist and Marxist analyses noted above). In addition, the highly ordered nature of the organization of medical practice itself intrinsically disallows major change other than under the most extreme circumstances. Only when problems appear beyond solution, given present tools and practices, and when the demand for their resolution becomes overwhelming, is major change likely to occur.

What is much more likely to happen when a paradigm community is faced with a variety of initially unresolvable problems is the development of minor modifications that will somehow mitigate the problems or make them seem less in need of total resolution. These modifications may be no more extensive than the typical incrementalism (or muddling through, cf. Lindblom, 1959) that occurs in the "normal" growth of paradigm practices noted above. However, the modifications may be more significant in that: (1) they are a minor break from existing patterns of practice, and (2) they may be highlighted because of their potential for resolving problems that are already in the limelight. Such is the case with American health care today.

There are extensive changes occurring in American health care -- extensive in the sense that they appear in many different segments of health care and that they occupy considerable attention of policymakers and others -- yet none of those changes, taken singly or as a whole, are necessarily of great significance. They do not challenge the fundamental organizational/political arrangements that have existed for some time, nor do they challenge the basic assumptions or practices of the dominant health care paradigm.

The "radical critics" may thus be correct in predicting that there will be no changes that will greatly alter the present system. But they are incorrect to argue that no changes can occur. The most important question is the extent to which the changes that can occur may make a difference in the health care received by the American public. But to ask this question one must ask two further questions: Who judges what constitutes "making a difference"? and What are the criteria used in making that judgement?

Even if we had answers to the two questions just posed, contemporary social scientists and policy makers would still be faced with a range of potential differences in how to view the current situation in health care and in the conclusions that can be drawn. The chapters in this volume reflect that diversity.

POLICY DEVELOPMENT AND THE ASSESSMENT OF CHANGE

Let us examine the professionals and organizations that constitute at least part of the membership of the paradigm community, for they are most likely to be involved in issues of assessment and policy development. A number of rather striking characteristics can be noted. First, during a crisis period, evaluation becomes a paramount concern. If a health care organization is challenged as not meeting the needs of its clients - that is, if it is accused of being a part of "the problem" - it will want evidence to refute such challenges or it will accept the allegations as accurate and attempt to implement changes. In either case, the organization will need data to support its present activities or to evaluate and justify newly instituted changes. (Other obvious scenarios are also possible, but all tend to involve significant use of evaluation.)

Second, the formulation of policy comes to the fore as a concomitant concern. In "normal times" policymaking is a necessary activity to maintain both order and accountability. In crisis times, effective policymaking, presumably based upon careful evaluation, is seen as the primary means of solving problems and eliminating the crisis. Policymaking itself may even become more important to participants than the activities that prompted the policy formulation (cf. Lindbolm and Cohen, 1979).

Third, given that the paradigm is at least temporarily unsuccessful in accomplishing the things it is supposed to, the paradigm's links with the larger society will be potentially threatened, the legitimacy of the paradigm could be called into question, and there is always the chance that such questioning will undermine its links with the larger society, thereby encouraging the development of an alternative paradigm. And, where these links are ones of funding, as is the case in health care, the threat may be seen as very significant indeed. Under such conditions -- which might reasonably be argued to exist in U.S. health care today -- the organization will not only be preeminently concerned with evaluation and policymaking but may also be concerned with maintaining legitimacy in the public, or more specifically, the governmental eye, than in using evaluation to find a solution that might eventually eliminate the crisis (cf. Meyer and Rowan, 1977; Imershein et al., 1981; Imershein, 1980). Thus health care organizations may seek evaluations, policies, and reform commissions that will provide results consistent with public expectations, particularly those of funding sources. Whether any of these activities have positive effect on the continuing problems that are ostensibly their focus may become a secondary concern at best (contrast this with Alford's analysis, 1975: Ch 2). I do not wish to imply that such organizations are willfully devious (although that may be true on occasion). Rather, I am suggesting that the preeminent requirements of the organizations' continuation are legitimacy and funding, and the problem-solving demanded by the crisis will simply be subsumed under those more immediate demands.

Thus, the consideration of "what makes a difference" may be very important for organizations seeking continued funding and legitimacy in a time of crisis; however, what they publically declare to be important may depend more on the "myths" expected by the public than on anything else (Meyer and Rowan, 1977; Imershein, 1980). To the extent that government reports depend upon information provided by such organizations or that social science research takes as given the data supplied by the organizations, judgements of what changes are significant will quite possibly be biased.

Turning specifically to the social science arena and to the chapters in this book, "what makes a difference" varies considerably depending on the context of the research and on what analytical perspective is brought to bear on the changes under consideration. Like the organizations, social scientists concerned with an area in crisis focus especially on matters of policymaking and evaluation. Much social science work is conducted in direct collaboration with or at the behest and funding, directly or indirectly, of the organization(s) being studied. In such cases, the research is likely to be characterized by some of the conditions noted above. And where the government (including funding agencies) relies extensively on information supplied from the organizations in question, the availability of research funds is likely to be similarly constrained, that is, the organizations will focus on studies that conform to current expectations and confirm the legitimacy of the organizations and their efforts at change. Since much research requires government funding as an essential resource, any review of research on areas in crisis, as in health care, must keep these potential "structural" limitations in mind. Marxist analyses that question the legitimacy of the entire health care system, for example, are less likely to be funded.

Much "evaluation" research (especially research sponsored by the organization being studied) and thus the bulk of research in the health arena is necessarily programmatic in nature and takes for granted the assumptions and goals of the organization under study. "What makes a difference" in this case is obviously attuned to the needs of the organization.

Nonetheless, some research does address such concerns from other perspectives, and substantive issues not tied to the immediate goals of an organization or service do get examined. The papers in this volume are a case in point. The majority of them are concerned in some fashion with organizational innovations in the health arena, but they address these changes from a critical perspective (such as the Marxist viewpoint) or with regard to a substantive issue (such as professional prestige or autonomy), that is not directly tied to organizational goals.

In sum, we can easily see how broad the spectrum of potentially significant changes in health care really is. Innovations have emerged from a variety of sources, usually in response to some problem in the health arena. Lack of sufficient services has prompted the use of non-physicians. Relative lack of coordination and direction has resulted in the development of Health Systems

Agencies as regulatory groups. The lack of alternative service models and the idea that health maintenance organizations could promote preventive care while being cost effective have prompted federal sponsorship of HMOs. Neighborhood health centers have been established to better respond to the needs of underserved urban neighborhoods. Consumers have been added to directorial boards to promote system responsiveness. Models for a national health system are being sought. Physicians are becoming more open with their patients, including those who are dying. Chiropractic has become a more acceptable alternative mode of practice. Health education is now a central concern within the system, at least ideologically.

The range of assessments and perspectives presented here is equally broad. Non-physicians can be used under some circumstances to provide more services. HMO's can be developed without apparently compromising professional autonomy. Health education is a much more widespread concern. Chiropractic is becoming a more viable alternative. But we also find that neighborhood health centers may be only one example of how government programs limit services to and exploit the lower classes. The presence of consumers on policy boards may have little effect on increasing the responsiveness of the system. The much-touted VA system displays all too many problems; problems that a similarly designed national health system would likely face. Needless to say, it is difficult to draw any clear conclusions from reviewing this selection of problems and perspectives.

Why, then, is it useful to engage in this sort of review? First, it makes apparent in a concrete way the diversity of problems, programs, and perspectives; the lack of consensus; and the difficulty of drawing conclusions regarding "what makes a difference." Second, it demonstrates the continuing concern within the field for these issues, and the unwillingness of social science researchers to rest with either of the more extreme positive or negative commentaries on the American health care system. Equally important, the diversity found in this book is representative of the larger process of paradigm crisis and reconsideration that pervades the health care system, and indicates the differing degrees of public commitment to or rejection of the current paradigm. The data do not and cannot "speak for themselves." They are described and understood from perspectives within the paradigm, critical of the paradigm, or completely outside the paradigm. The continuing process of change is inherently a political process, and this volume is both an instance of and a commentary on that process.

12

REFERENCES

Alford, Robert R.
    1975   Health Care Politics: Ideological and
            Interest Group Barriers to Reform. Chicago:
            University of Chicago Press.
Anderson, Odin W.
    1972   Health Care: Can There Be Equity? New York:
            Wiley.
Citizens Board of Inquiry into Health Services for
        Americans
    1972   Heal Yourself. Washington: American Public
            Health Association.
Ehrenreich, Barbara and John
    1970   The American Health Empire. New York: Random
            House.
Garfield, Sidney R.
    1970   "The Delivery of Medical Care." Scientific
            American 222 (April): 15-23.
Imershein, Allen W.
    1977a   "The Epistemological Bases of Social Order:
            Toward Ethnoparadigm Analysis." Ch. 1 (pp.
            1-51) in David Heise (ed.), Sociological
            Methodology 1977. Washington: Jossey-Bass.
    1977b   "Organizational Change as a Paradigm Shift."
            Sociological Quarterly 18 (Winter): 33-43.
    1980   "Reform and Legitimacy in Organizational
            Decision-Making." Paper presented at the
            annual meeting of the Midwest Sociological
            Society.
Imershein, Allen W., Michael Frumkin, Richard Chackerian,
        and Gerald McDonald
    1981   "A Critical Research Framework for Assessing
            Services Integration in Large, Human
            Resource Agencies." Evaluation and Change.
Kuhn, Thomas
    1977   "Institutionalized Organizations: Formal
            Structure as Myth and Ceremony." American
            Journal of Sociology 83 (No. 2):340-363.
Lindblom, Charles E.
    1959   "The Science of Muddling Through." Public
            Administration Review Vol. 19 (Spring): 79-88.
Linblom, Charles E. and David Cohen
    1979   Usable Knowledge. New Haven: Yale University
            Press.
Meyer, John W. and Brian Rowan
    1977   "Institutionalized Organizations: Formal
            Structure as Myth and Ceremony." American
            Journal of Sociology 83 (No. 2): 340-363.
Navarro, Vicente
    1976   Medicine Under Capitalism. New York: Prodist.
Schwartz, Harry
    1971   "Health Care in America: A Heretical
            Diagnosis." Saturday Review (August 14):
            14-17, 55.

2
The Public and Care by Non-Physicians: Health Policy Consideration

Bebe F. Lavin   Kent State University

In an effort to resolve what some define as a crisis in health care, medical paraprofessionals have become an increasing part of the primary care scene. As the training and use of paraprofessionals expands there has been growing insistence that much of what office-based physicians do could be handled as well or better by these non-physicians. If it is health policy to encourage the use of paraprofessionals to alleviate the shortages and maldistribution of primary care doctors, acceptance of these personnel by the public is a critical issue. A study of the public in a Midwest area suggests considerable variability in willingness to accept a trained person other than a doctor to do several tasks usually considered within the domain of the physician. The findings show that the typical demographic and attitudinal variables do little to explain differences in public willingness to accept paraprofessionals. However, the context in which service is delivered is suggested as a possible explanation of acceptance. Several policy relevant issues are discussed, including the need to provide settings for medical care that will maximize public willingness to be treated by non-physicians.

One solution to what some have defined as the crisis in the delivery of health care in the United States has been the redefinition and reallocation of tasks among the providers of primary care. Non-physician personnel are

This research was supported in part by U.S. Public Health Service Grant No. RO1-45-0849, National Center for Health Services Research. I acknowledge with gratitude the help of Marie Haug with this study and also thank those colleagues who commented on an earlier draft of this article when presented at the annual meeting of the Society for the Study of Social Problems, Boston, 1979.

trained increasingly to handle many of the wide range of problems now presented to primary care doctors. In particular persons titled nurse practitioners, physicians' assistants, nurse extenders, or ancillary health workers are expected to act in concert with physicians to provide the basic health and illness care needed by the vast majority of people who seek medical attention.

It has been estimated that 60 percent of patient visits to physicians are for general or primary care (Rogers, 1977), while perhaps 75 to 80 percent of all requests made in primary care settings could be taken care of by the appropriately trained nurse practitioner (Mauksh, 1978). Cohen (Cohen et al., 1974) suggests that at least 66 percent of the patients seen by midlevel practitioners can be managed with no consultation with physicians. Although there is nothing extraordinary about doctors' use of personnel to assist in the varied tasks of their practice, the different and current implication is that much of what office-based primary care physicians do could be handled as well as or better by a non-physician. A recent article in a well-know medical journal establishes this theme in the title by asking, "Does the Practice of Medicine Require a Medical Degree?" (Sox, 1978).

The issue of the expanded use of non-physicians in primary care is raised in several contexts. For example, use of such manpower is a means to alleviate the perceived maldistribution and/or shortage of primary care doctors (Eisenberg, 1977; Rogers, 1977). Moreover, it affords economies by making better use of the time of a high priced commodity, the physician (Margulies, 1975; Nelson et al., 1975). Further, it is suggested that expansion in knowledge and technology, along with the need to integrate the varied and often non-medical problems that patients bring to physicians, require specialization and a new division of labor (Bates, 1970; Breslau, 1977; Svarstad, 1976; Thomas, 1977).

Although most of the programs for the training and utilization of these midlevel practitioners have been in existence for a relatively short period of time--ten to fifteen years--a growing body of literature has developed. Many of the more recent studies focus on the problems of appropriate role definitions (Barr, 1978; Burkett et al., 1978; Mauksch and Young, 1974, Merenstein et al., 1974; Record and Greenlick, 1973) and different patterns of use as related to client characteristics (Duttera and Harlan, 1978; Herman, 1972; Hessel and Haggerty, 1968; Lewis et al., 1976; Morris and Smith, 1977; Roemer, 1976).

Perhaps the most critical issues, however, have not been adequately addressed. The first is the question of the quality of the care by non-physicians, the second is the willingness of the public to accept such personnel.

Quality of care is an elusive concept and is difficult to measure (Kissick, 1971). Nevertheless numerous studies have attempted to assess quality of non-physician services. A comprehensive review of this research through 1975 (Celentano, 1978) reveals that the methodologies of this type of research are deficient--a problem noted by others as well (Sox, 1978). In order to accept the findings of studies which conclude that the quality of care by midlevel practitioners is as safe and as effective as the care provided by a physician (Cohen et al., 1974; Tompkins et al., 1977; Sackett et al., 1974; Spitzer et al., 1974), one needs to ignore such criticism of methodologies. However, none of this research links the use of paraprofessionals to the two-class nature of the health care system (Krause, 1977). Some writers have implied that the poor, ghetto residents and rural patients, those most often treated by non-physicians, could be receiving second class medical treatment or at least they may view it as such (Rushing and Miles, 1977).

This leads to the second major question. What is the degree to which the public is willing to accept the non-physician in lieu of the doctor? The answers to this are few, and do not reflect consensus because they are often based on anecdotal studies of limited generalizability (Pickard, 1976). For example, some studies report that patient acceptance of non-physicians and patient satisfaction with care is at a high level (Breslau, 1977; Greenfield et al., 1975; Lewis, 1971; Linn, 1975; Pondy, 1970). Yet, Andersen (1971) found the public is reluctant to allow non-physicians to do some common and not technically difficult medical tasks.

An opportunity to examine public response to non-physicians became available in connection with a study primarily concerned with the examination of the authority relationship between physicians and the public (Haug and Lavin, 1977). The data collected in that study allowed assessment of the degree to which the public is willing to accept the use of trained persons other than a physician to perform certain patient care tasks which are ordinarily considered the domain of the physician. Further, the data explored demographic and attitudinal factors which might explain differences in acceptance.

STUDY SETTING AND METHODS

The data reported here are based on a survey of the public, using a randomly selected sample from three different sized Midwest communities during Spring, 1976. Person-to-person interviews lasting nearly an hour were conducted by trained interviewers. A response rate of 82 percent yielded 640 cases for analysis. As compared with census data on the total population, older and better educated persons are somewhat over-represented, but in general the study sample is typical of the American public.

In order to measure acceptance of paraprofessionals, the public sampled was asked how willing they would be to let some trained person other than a doctor do the following tasks:

1. give shots;
2. advise on routine problems;
3. do a routine physical exam;
4. deliver babies;
5. prescribe medicines;
6. remove tonsils.

The items are presented here in the order which emerged in a Guttman analysis, rather than the order used in the interview. Although the Guttman analysis (Nie et al., 1975) did not quite reach acceptable scalability criteria (coefficient of reproducibility of .87 and coefficient of scalability of .55), it was useful in drawing attention to the order of "difficulty" in accepting the items. Thus 84 percent of the respondents would be willing to have non-physicians give shots, and almost 60 percent would accept advice on routine problems or allow a paraprofessional to do a routine physical. Nearly half would be willing to use a non-physician to deliver a baby. However only about 16 percent would allow trained paraprofessionals to prescribe medicine or remove tonsils.

For the purposes of this report a summated index of Acceptance of Medical Paraprofessionals was used. A rejection of any item was scored as one, a qualified yes as two, and an unqualified yes as three. The summated total was then divided by the number of items answered. In effect this meant that if any items were not answered, a score was equal to the mean of the other answers of that respondent. To avoid fractional numbers, all were multiplied by ten. Thus the dependent variable, Acceptance of Medical Paraprofessionals, had a theoretical range of ten to thirty, with the higher score indicative of higher acceptance.

Certain variables seem likely to affect public willingness to accept other than a doctor to do certain tasks and therefore are included as explanatory. The authority of physicians, and thereby the legitimation of the definition of the tasks they consider a part of their role, rests in the expectation that they have greater knowledge and expertise than do other health personnel or patients. Also, their authority derives from the expectation that their overriding concern is for what is best for their patients (Parsons, 1951, 1975; Gill, 1978). It could then be anticipated that to the degree that the public is knowledgeable about health matters or to the extent that they doubt the expertise or the concern of the physician, legitimation of the authority of the physician will be called into question. This, in turn, will increase the likelihood for the acceptance of others in the doctor's role. Accordingly, level of health knowledge is introduced as a major explanatory variable, along with five psychosocial variables that were expected to indicate the public's attitudes about either medicine in general or doctors in particular.

A scale measuring skepticism of medicine and of doctors developed in earlier research (Suchman, 1965), indicates whether respondents doubt the efficacy of medicine or the ability of doctors to cure their ills. The belief in physicians' competence or the belief in doctors' personal concern for patients was assessed by the scale created originally by Zyzanski and colleagues (Zyzanski et al., 1974). Finally a measure of willingness to question doctors' authority was developed from the Adorno F-Scale (Roginson and Shaver, 1973.)[1] For each of these attitude variables, in which the direction suggested less belief in either medicine or doctors or in which questions were raised as to the physician's authority in medical encounters, it was anticipated that there would be greater willingness to accept trained non-physicians.

The demographic characteristics of age and social class are included not only because they may reflect differences in levels of education but also because younger, middle class, and by implication better educated, persons could be expected to take a more challenging attitude toward physicians (Haug and Lavin, 1978). Moreover, good health and little experience with doctors and medical settings were expected to indicate low dependency on physicians and therfore greater acceptance of the use of non-physicians. Race, sex, and level of urbanization were other demographic variables included since their effects on other health behaviors have been previously noted. For purposes of analysis, level of knowledge is also considered a demographic characteristic.

FINDINGS

The findings reveal considerable variability in this public's willingness to accept a trained person other than a doctor to do the several tasks suggested (Table 2.1). When scores are grouped, the distribution approaches the normal, with the mean of nearly 19, and a standard deviation of 5. But it must be noted that about 26 percent reject allocating most of these tasks to

---

[1]For further description of this variable, see Haug and Lavin (1978).

paraprofessionals, while less than 14 percent are in the
two highest categories, indicating that few accept the
use of non-physicians for all or nearly all of these
health care activities.

TABLE 2.1
Willingness to Accept Medical Paraprofessionals (percents)

Score	Percent
10-12 (low)	12.0
13-14	14.0
16-18	21.4
19-20	19.8
22-24	19.2
25-27	8.0
28-30 (high)	5.6
TOTAL	100.0
N	637
$\overline{X}$	18.9
SD	5.3

In order to evaluate to what extent any of the
demographic or attitudinal variables could explain the
differences found in Acceptance of Medical Paraprofessionals, zero-order correlations and stepwise multiple
regessions were calculated. Four of the demographic
variables--health knowledge, age, sex, and social class,
and two of the attitudes--belief in physician competence
and a questioning of physician authority, are statistically significant at the zero-order level. This finding
indicates that the relationship of these variables to
Acceptance of Medical Paraprofessionals is not due to
sampling error (Table 2.2, column A). Those respondents
with greater health knowledge, younger, male, or of
higher social class were more likely to show a greater
willingness to accept non-physicians. However the correlations are substantively small. Health knowledge, the
most important variable, explains only a little over 5
percent of the variance. At the social psychological
level, those willing to question the doctor's authority
were willing to accept "surrogate" doctors. Contrary to
expectations, those with a high belief in doctors' competency were also willing to accept such care. Both of
these correlations were at statistically significant but
substantively trivial levels.
In the stepwise multiple regression, all the

TABLE 2.2
Relationship of Selected Demographic and Social
Psychological Variables to Willingness to Accept Medical
Paraprofessionals

	A Simple r	B[1] Beta
Demographic		
Health knowledge	.233*	.18*
Sex	-.146*	-.15*
Family Social Class	.177*	.09*
Age	-.123*	-.09*
Race	.043	
Level of Urbanization	.018	
Health status	.045	
Medical experience	-.057	
Social Psychological		
Belief in doctor competence	.116*	.10*
Questioning doctor authority	.126*	
Belief in doctor concern	.038	
Skepticism of doctors	.011	
Skepticism of medicine	-.051	

R^2 = .11 $F_{13,589}$ = 5.44 $p < .001$

*statistically significant at .05 level or better

[1]B refers to standardized regression coefficients, beta, and are reported only if they met the F or tolerance level (F = 1.5, T = .50).

---

theoretically meaningful variables were entered into the same equation whether or not they were statistically significant at the zero order level. This procedure reveals the impact of each of the explanatory variables on the dependent variable when all others are taken into account and uses beta weights as the criteria for relative importance. Now only five of the entire set are statistically significant--health knowledge, age, sex, social class, and belief in doctors' competency. Questioning doctors' authority does not emerge as occuring beyond chance (Table 2.2, column B). The most salient variables in the explanation of willingness to accept non-physicians are greater health knowledge (Beta = .18), being male (Beta = -.15), believing in physician competence (Beta = .10), higher social class (Beta = .09), and younger age (Beta = -.09). Although the coefficient of determination is statistically significant, this variable set explains only 11 percent of the variance, suggesting that other factors are at work.

In order to explore these relationships further, the analysis was repeated for each individual item making up the Acceptance of Medical Paraprofessionals scale. The results reveal two distinctly different patterns (Table 2.3). One set of four items, (Give Shots, Advise on Routine Problems, Do a Routine Physical Exam, and Deliver Babies) shows a pattern somewhat similar to the total scale. The R^2s are not markedly different, ranging from .06 to .13, and except for Advise on Routine Problems, the most important explanatory variables emerging from the stepwise regression continue to be health knowledge and sex. It is noteworthy that these are the same tasks that members of the public might have observed paraprofessionals performing in doctors' offices, clinics or hospitals during previous visits.

Two other items, Prescribe Medicines and Remove Tonsils, are left almost completely unexplained by the independent variables utilized--R^2 is .01 in each case--, and health knowledge disappears from the regression. It is noteworthy in this instance that the two tasks mentioned are not performed currently by paraprofessionals, and are highly unlikely to have been experienced previously by the public. Unfortunately the data are not available for testing the effect on acceptance of past exposure to paraprofessional services.

These findings would generally indicate the advisability of dropping the Prescription and Tonsils items from the scale, and recalculating the regression equations. However, examination of the point-biserial item to total correlations shows that these items have the highest correlation values (.61 and .63) and thus are not candidates for elimination on the basis of usual scale analysis criterion.

Another intriguing finding is that the effect of age is reversed on the Deliver Babies item. Here it is the older rather than the younger respondents who are willing to have a non-physician take this responsibility. Experience could be once again explanatory. Older generations may recall a time when midwives, not obstetricians, officiated at births and are comfortable with this state of affairs.

In sum, both the total scale and individual item analysis reveal that the postulated array of explanatory variables is incomplete and that other factors need to be identified. The item analysis suggests that at least one of these is past exposure to paraprofessionals at work.

TABLE 2.3
Relationship of Selected Demographic and Social Psychological Variables to the Six Items of Willingness to Accept Medical Paraprofessionals

	Give Shots		Advise Routine		Routine Exams		Deliver Babies		Prescribe Medicine		Remove Tonsils	
	r^1	b^2	r	b	r	b	r	b	r	b	r	b
Demographic												
Health knowledge	.291*	.23*	.222*	.20*	.123*	.09*	.165*	.17*	-.001		.033	
Sex	-.112*	-.10*	-.024		-.132	-.13*	-.159*	-.16*	-.037		-.095	.10*
Family Social Class	.181*	.05	.142*		.099*		.109*		.067	.08*	.034	
Age	-.073		-.155*	.123*	-.193*	-.18*	.089*	.13*	-.046		-.068	.07*
Race	.167*	.09*	-.019		-.006		.087*		-.035		-.017	
Level of Urbanization	.050		-.010		.019		.025		-.059	-.08*	.026	
Health status	.107*		-.014		.049		.017		-.005		-.021	
Medical experience	-.089*	-.07*	.015		-.070		-.016		.007		-.017	
Social Psychological												
Belief in doctor competence	.123*	.09	.034		.121*	.12*	.090*	.07*	.051		.026	
Questioning doctor authority	.138	.06	.120*		.086*		.065	.06	.013		.049	
Belief in doctor concern	.004		.037		.052		.038		.015		-.017	
Skepticism of doctors	.013		.052		-.015		-.011		.007		-.011	
Skepticism of medicine	-.037		-.021		-.055		-.015		.062	.064*	-.015	
R^2	.13		.08		.06		.08		.01		.01	
F	11.91		11.76		19.58		9.42		2.36		3.97	
	p<.01		p<.01		p<.01		p<.01		ns		p<.05	

[1]r refers to the simple, zero order correlation coefficient
[2]b refers to standardized regression coefficients, beta, and are reported only if they met the F or tolerance level (F=1.5, T=.50)
*statistically significant at .05 level or greater

DISCUSSION

These findings raise a number of difficult questions that have policy implications. First, why do health status, medical experience, and various attitudes about the efficacy of medicine and physicians have so little effect on willingness to use non-physicians, while belief in doctor's competence is, even if weakly, related? It might be due to a recognition among younger, more knowledgeable, and more middle class persons that most of the tasks involved are really not that complex or life threatening, and are generally done under a doctor's direction. And a competent doctor will monitor that they are done properly. Thus whether one's own health is good or bad, or one's view of medicine and medical care providers is skeptical or not is not as critical in acceptance as being knowledgeable about health matters. From a policy perspective, this suggests that programs of education can increase acceptance of paraprofessional use.

Second, is it likely that those most accepting will be those most apt to utilize paraprofessionals? Since the poor, black, elderly and rural populations suffer most from maldistributions of physicians, and thus are more often treated by paraprofessionals, the groups exposed to this type of care are in fact, found to be the most rejecting or indifferent. Race and level of urbanization were not relevant to acceptance. It was the older and lower social class respondents who were more likely to eschew paraprofessionals as less acceptable, perhaps viewing their use as providing second class care, continuing in a new form the discrimination they have suffered in the past. This suggests extension of policies that press physicians to practice in underserved areas, rather than emphasizing substitute care providers.

Thirdly, what factors are likely to account for the 90 percent or more of unexplained variance in this study? From a policy point of view, this is an important question. Assuming that health provider shortages and maldistributions will continue to be alleviated by training new types of paraprofessional labor, it will be important to uncover factors that encourage public acceptance. One factor not evaluated in this study that could be crucial is the degree to which the public accepts care by physicians and non-physicians as equivalent. Two recent studies of public attitude toward physicians' assistants and nurse practitioners indicate that the public does not judge care by non-physicians as equivalent to that of doctors. An important reservation made by these respondents is that such care be supervised by a physician (Litman, 1971; Storms and Fox, 1979). In the research reported in this article the public was asked about their willingness to accept a physician substitute, not an assistant. Findings suggest that their willingness to do so is, at least in part, the result of a realistic evaluation of medical tasks. Therefore, public acceptance of physician substitutes would necessitate reevaluation by the public of tasks customarily performed by physicians and require in many cases, a demystification of these tasks. Such prospects seem unlikely.

Another factor affecting public acceptance of non-physicians might be the response to potentially lower fees being charged by paraprofessionals for the same tasks performed by physicians. It is likely that any differences in fees would be interpreted as indicating a two-tiered system of health care. Those unable to select medical alternatives would then believe that they were in fact receiving second class medical care.

Thus a further question is raised as to the point of intervention in order to encourage broader public willingness to use non-physicians in primary care. Since the standard demographic variables function weakly if at all, while health status and attitudes are generally irrelevant to acceptance, these factors cannot be considered as change agents. As the individual item analysis indicated, the answer may involve differential exposure to the paraprofessionals who give service. However this creates a logical dilemma. If the poor, black, elderly and rural are most apt to be treated by non-physicians, and thus are most experienced with this type of care, why are they not also the most accepting? Could it be that their lack of alternative sources of care forces acceptance as a matter of necessity rather than choice, and creates thereby a sense of deprivation and negative feelings?

In other words, the conditions under which the experience occurs is critical. In the context of superior care, usually the case for patients of higher social class, paraprofessionals are acceptable as physician extenders once their services have been experienced. In the context of episodic and less-superior care, usually the case for disadvantaged patients, paraprofessionals are less acceptable as physician substitutes, and may appear to symbolize deprivation. Thus there is an interaction between the experience of paraprofessional care and the quality of the circumstances in which that care is delivered.

Accordingly, from a policy perspective, one might suggest that improving the quality and context of health services are necessary preconditions for extending acceptance of the use of non-physicians in the delivery of medical care. Unfortunately current policy decisions seem to be based on speculation and guesswork about public reaction. This can lead to the creation of more problems than the ones the policy makers are attempting to resolve.

REFERENCES

Andersen, Ronald
    1971   "The Public's View of the Crisis in Medical
            Care: An Impetus for Changing Delivery
            Systems?" Economic and Business Bulletin 24
            (Fall):44-52.
Barr, Judith K.
    1978   "The Health Associate: Definition of a New
            Role."   Paper   presented   at   the   Eastern
            Sociological Society, Philadelphia (April).
Bates, Barbara
    1970   "Doctor   and   Nurse: Changing   Roles   and
            Relations." New England Journal of Medicine.
            283:129-134.
Breslau, Naomi
    1977   "The Role of the Nurse-Practitioner in a
            Pediatric   Team: Patient   Definitions."
            Medical Care 15 (December):1014-23.
Burkett, Gaye L., Margaret Parken-Harris, Joan C. Kuhn
            and Gerald H. Escovitz
    1978   "A Comparative Study of Physicians and Nurses'
            Conceptions of the Role of Nurse Practi-
            tioner."   American Journal of Public Health
            68 (November): 1090-95.
Celentano, David D.
    1978   "Critical Policy Issues Concerning New Health
            Practitioners--Quality of Care."   Sociologi-
            cal Symposium 23 (Summer):61-77.
Cohen, E.D., L.M. Crootof, M.G. Goldfarb, K. Keenen, M.
            Korper and M. Triffin
    1974   An Evaluation of Policy Related Research on
            New and Expanded Roles of Health Workers.
            New   Haven,   Conn.:   Office   of   Regional
            Activities and Continuing Education, Yale
            University School of Medicine.
Duttera,   Julian   M.   and   William   R.   Harlan
    1978   "Evaluation of Physician Assistants in Rural
            Primary   Care."   Archives   of   Internal
            Medicine 138 (February):224-28.
Eisenberg, Leon
    1977   "The Search for Care." Daedalus 106 (Winter):
            235-45.
Gill, Derek G.
    1978   "Limitation upon Choice and Constraints Over
            Decision-Making in Doctor/Patient Exchanges."
            Pp. 141-154 in Eugene Gallagher (ed.) The
            Doctor-Patient Relationship in the Changing
            Health Scene: An International Perspective.
            Washington,   D.C.:   John   E.   Fogarty
            International Center for Advanced Study in the
            Health Sciences.

Greenfield, S., F.E. Bragg, D.L. McCraith, and J.
    Blackburn
    1975   "Upper-Respiratory Tract Complaint Protocol
             for Physician-Extenders." Archives of
             Internal Medicine, 133:294-99.
Haug, Marie and Bebe Lavin
    1977   Final Report: Public Challenge to MD
             Authority. U.S. Public Health Grant
             #1-R01-HS-0849-01.
    1978   "Method of Payment for Medical Care and
             Patient Attitudes to Physician Authority."
             Journal of Health and Social Behavior.
             19(September):279-291.
Herman, Mary W.
    1972   "The Poor: Their Medical Needs and the
             Health Services Available to Them." The
             Annals (January):12-21.
Hessel, Samuel J. and Robert J. Haggerty
    1968   "General Pediatrics: A Study of Practices
             in the Mid-1960s." Journal of Pediatrics 2
             (August):271-79.
Kissick, William L
    1971   "Health Manpower in Transition." Pp. 162-
             206 in Ray Elling (ed.) National Health
             Care: Issues and Problems in Socialized
             Medicine. New York: Aldine-Atherton.
Krause, Elliott A.
    1977   Power and Illness: The Political Sociology
             of Health and Medical Care. New York:
             Elsevier, North Holland, Inc.
Lewis, Charles E.
    1971   "The Efficiency of New Health Manpower." A
             paper presented at the Invitational Health
             Services Research Conference. Chicago,
             Illinois (December).
Lewis, Charles E., Rashi Fein, and David Mechanic
    1976   A Right to Health. New York: John Wiley
             and Sons.
Linn, Lawrence S.
    1975   "Factors Associated with Patient Evaluation
             of Health Care." Health and Society
             53:531-548.
Litman, T.J.
    1972   "Public Perception of the Physicians'
             Assistant - A Survey of the Attitudes and
             Opinions of Rural Iowa and Minnesota
             Residents." American Journal of Public
             Health 62:343.
Margulies, H.
    1975   Final Report of the Physician Extender Work
             Group. Washington, D.C.: Health Resource
             Administration, U.S. Department of Health,
             Education and Welfare.

26

Mauksch, Ingebor G.
    1978   "The Nurse Practitioner Movement--Where Does
                It Go from Here?"   American Journal of
                Public Health 68 (November):1074-75.
Mauksch, Ingebor G. and P.R. Young
    1974   "Nurse-Physician Interaction in a Family
                Medical Care Center."   Nursing Outlook
                22:113-119.
Merenstein, J.J., H. Wolfe and K.M. Barker
    1974   "The Use of Nurse Practitioners in General
                Practice." Medical Care 12:445-452.
Morris, Stephen B. and David B. Smith
    1977   "The Distribution of Physician Extenders."
                Medical Care 15 (December):1045-57.
Nelson, E.C., A.R. Jacobs, P.E. Breen and K.G. Johnson
    1975   "Impact of Physician's Assistant on Patient
                Visits   in   Ambulatory   Care   Practices."
                Annals   of   Internal   Medicine   82:608-612.
Nie, Norman H., C. Hadlai, Jean Jenkins, Karin
            Steinbrenner, and Dale Brent
    1975   Statistical Package for the Social Sciences,
                2nd edition. New York: McGraw-Hill.
Parsons, Talcott
    1951   The Social System.   Glencoe: Free Press.
    1975   "The Sick Role and the Role of the Physician
                Reconsidered."   Milbank Memorial Fund
                Quarterly, Health and Society 53:257-278.
Pickard, Glen C., Jr.
    1976   "Midlevel   Practitioners: Nurse   Practi-
                tioners and Physicians' Assistants."   Pp.
                129-140 in John Noble (ed.) Primary Care and
                the Practice of Medicine. Boston: Little,
                Brown and Company.
Pondy, Louis
    1970   "A Study of Patient Acceptance of Physi-
                cian's Assistant."   Durham, N.C.:   Duke
                University, GBSA Paper no. 27.
Record, Jane C. and Merwyn R. Greenlick
    1973   "New Health Professionals and Physician Role:
                An Hypothesis from Kaiser Experience."
                Public Health Reports 90(May):241-246.
Robinson, John and Phillip R. Shaver
    1973   Measures of Social Psychological Attitudes.
                Revised   Edition.   Ann   Arbor: Survey
                Research   Center,   Institute   for   Social
                Research: 308-317.
Roemer, Milton I.
    1976   Rural Health Care.   St. Louis: C.V. Mosby.
Rogers, David E.
    1977   "The Challenge of Primary Care."   Daedalus
                106 (Winter):81-105.

Rushing, William A. and David L. Miles
    1977   "Physicians, Physicians' Assistants, and the
                Social   Characteristics   of   Patients   in
                Southern   Appalachia."   Medical   Care   15
                (December):1004-1013
Sackett, D.L., W.O. Spitzer, M. Gent and R.S. Roberts
    1974   "The   Burlington   Randomized   Trial   of   the
                Nurse Practitioners: Health Outcomes of
                Patients."   Annals of Internal Medicine 80
                (2):137-142.
Sox, Harold C., Jr.
    1978   "Does the Practice of Medicine Require a
                Medical   Degree?"   Archives   of   Internal
                Medicine 138 (February):199-200.
Spitzer, W.O., E.D. Sackett, J.C. Sibley, R.S. Roberts,
        M. Gent, D.J. Kergen, B.C. Hackett and A.
        Olynick
    1974   "The   Burlington   Randomized   Trial   of   the
                Nurse Practitioner." New England Journal of
                Medicine 290-251.
Storms, Doris M. and John G. Fox
    1979   "The Public's View of Physicians' Assistants
                and   Nurse   Practitioners: A   Survey   of
                Baltimore Urban Residents." Medical Care 17
                (May): 526-535.
Suchman, Edward A.
    1965   "Social   Patterns   of   Illness   and   Medical
                Care." Journal of Health and Human Behavior
                6(Fall): 115-128.
Svarstad, Bonnie L.
    1976   "Physician-Patient Communication and Patient
                Conformity with Medical Advice."   Pp. 220-
                238 in David Mechanic (ed.), The Growth
                of   Bureaucratic   Medicine.   New   York:
                Wiley-Interscience.
Thomas, Lewis
    1977   "On the Science and Technology of Medicine."
                Daedalus 106(Winter):35-47.
Tompkins, Richard, Robert Wood, Barry Wolcott, B. Timothy
        Walsh
    1977   "The   Effectiveness   and   Cost   of   Acute
                Respiratory Illness Medical Care Provided by
                Physicians and Algorithm-Assisted
                Physicians'   Assistants."   Medical   Care
                15(December):991-1003.
Zyzanski, S.J., B.S. Hulka and J.C. Cassel
    1974   "Scale for the Measurement of 'Satisfaction'
                with Medical Care: Modifications in Con-
                tent, Format and Scoring."   Medical Care
                12:611-20.

3
Organizational Structure and Professional Norms in an Alternative Health Care Setting: Physicians in Health Maintenance Organizations

Judith K. Barr   Rutgers University, Newark
Marcia K. Steinberg   Rider College

The development of new organizational forms for the delivery of health and medical care in the U.S. includes health maintenance organizations (HMOs), designed to provide a set of comprehensive basic health services to a defined population for a fixed prepaid premium. As complex organizations, HMOs have the potential for limiting the autonomy of professionals working in them. This paper describes the legal requirements and organizational mechanisms under which physicians practice in HMOs and considers the potential for conflict between the organization and professional norms.

On the basis of document and interview data from nine HMOs, it appears that mechanisms developed to implement the mode of physician reimbursement and legal requirements for quality assurance and member grievance procedures do not limit physician autonomy in these HMOs. Variation was observed among the three organizational models: staff, group, and independent practice association.

INTRODUCTION

It has recently been argued that a variety of societal forces are combining to challenge the position of the medical profession and erode professional autonomy and control over conditions of practice. These forces include increasing bureaucratization and government

---

A version of this paper was presented at the Annual Meeting of the Society for the Study of Social Problems, Boston, August, 1979. The senior author appreciates the helpful comments of Louis H. Orzack and Ralph Larkin on an earlier draft. This research was supported in part by a grant from the Applied Social Research Coordinating Council, Rutgers University, Newark.

intervention, as well as rising levels of consumer education and interest (Haug, 1976; Child and Schriesheim,
1978). One potential source of challenge lies in alternative ways of organizing medical practice and the delivery of services which have been developed as part of the
response to problems in the health care system in the
United States.

Among these alternative forms of health care delivery are health maintenance organizations (HMOs), designed
to provide a set of comprehensive basic health services to
a voluntarily enrolled population for a fixed, prepaid
premium. Within this concept, a variety of organizational
structures is possible, and different arrangements for
the delivery of care have emerged with physicians providing services under varying modes of reimbursement.
The purposes of this paper are to describe the organizational arrangements and legal requirements under which
physicians practice in HMOs, to report empirical evidence
about the implementation of these structural elements,
and to consider the potential for strain between organizational requirements and professional norms.

THEORETICAL BACKGROUND

A considerable body of literature postulates a clash
between the colleague control structures of professions
and the system of hierarchical control characteristic of
complex organizations (Blau and Scott, 1961; Etzioni,
1961; Thompson, 1961). Scott (1966:269) suggests that
professionals may resist bureaucratic rules, reject
bureaucratic standards, resist bureaucratic supervision
and give limited, conditional loyalty to the organization.
Various accommodative mechanisms have been identified
which limit strain between professional norms and
bureaucratic requirements (Litwak, 1961; Scott, 1966).
Barber (1963) notes the existence of differentiated role
structures for carrying out professional work partially
separated from the organization as a whole and differentiated authority structures in which professionals serve
as administrators. Goss (1961) found that hospital clinic physicians accepted hierarchical authority exercised
by physician administrators over administrative matters,
while maintaining their individual authority over patient
care activities within a framework of advisory relationships with physicians.

How professionals respond in organizational settings
has been linked to various characteristics of the organization. In his comparative study of occupations, Hall
(1968) found that professionalization and bureaucratization were inversely related so that perceptions of autonomy were negatively related to hierarchy of authority,
division of labor, formal procedures, and impersonality.
The generalization that the maintenance of professional

norms varies with the level of bureaucratization of the setting has been supported in the health field. Engel (1969) observed that perceived autonomy among physicians varied with three types of bureaucratic settings: solo or small group practice (non-bureaucratic), a privately owned closed-panel medical organization (moderately bureaucratic), and a governmental medical organization (highly bureaucratic). Physicians in the moderately-bureaucratic setting perceived the greatest autonomy with respect to their professional work; Engel concluded that there may be an optimal level of bureaucracy in which limits on autonomy are balanced by factors which facilitate professionals' goals.

Freidson (1970) has argued that autonomy is the core characteristic of a profession, that physicians have exclusive rights over medical practice, and that medical practice has been organized to facilitate physician autonomy and control.[1] Larson (1977) has recently argued that professions and organizations are both part of a process of rationalization of work; therefore, they may be seen as complementary rather than conflicting modes of organizing work. From another perspective, professions are seen as composed of segmented interest groups moving at different rates to maximize various "professional" characteristics (Bucher and Strauss, 1961). In this view, autonomy is not considered an attribute which necessarily accompanies the functioning of a professional (Roth, 1974). Rather, this concept is an important dimension regarding professionals in work settings which can be studied under varying conditions (Nathanson and Becker, 1972; Madison, et al., 1977).

From any of these perspectives, the extent of professional autonomy in bureaucratic settings can be considered problematic. As complex organizations, HMOs are one context in which this issue can be studied.

HEALTH MAINTENANCE ORGANIZATIONS

The term health maintenance organizations was first described in 1970 (Ellwood, et al., 1971). It incorporated group practice concepts and prepayment within a new structural form for the delivery of comprehensive ambulatory health care. HMOs were intended to address a

---

[1]That these two concepts are empirically, as well as conceptually, distinct has been demonstrated in the work of Nathanson and Becker (1972). Following their distinction, autonomy is defined as freedom from non-professional determination and evaluation of work activities, whereas control is defined as influence over organizational policies and the work of non-professionals.

variety of problems, including high costs and lack of accessibility, and to promote consumer accountability and quality of care. The Federal HMO Act (P.L. 93-222) of 1973 was the first effort to put this concept into law. According to the legislation, an HMO is an organized system for the delivery of a set of comprehensive health and medical services under a contractual arrangement with a voluntarily enrolled population for a fixed prepaid premium which is the HMO's major source of revenue.

In the 1976 amendments (P.L. 94-460) to the law, three organizational models are delineated, all operating under the prepayment mechanism but differentiated by practice site and mode of physician reimbursement (U.S. Department of Health, Education, and Welfare, 1977). These three models are:

1. Staff: central facility; physicians are salaried employees of the HMO.
2. Group: central facility; physicians are part of a medical group, partnership, or corporation reimbursed by salary or capitation[2] through the group.
3. IPA (Individual Practice Association): physicians practice in their private offices; physicians are part of partnership, corporation, or association which contracts with the HMO; and they are reimbursed individually on a fee-for-service basis through the medical group.[3]

The federal HMO law also sets guidelines and regulations which embody organizational requirements that may affect physicians and the way they practice. Ongoing quality assurance programs must be established to assure maintenance of standards and high quality in both the process and outcomes of care; such programs must ensure the HMO meets standards for hospitalization set up by physicians on a community basis. The law also requires that there be "meaningful" procedures for hearing and resolving grievances by HMO members, providing a mechanism for member complaints about services or other problems.

---

[2]Capitation refers to a specified amount paid per enrollee for a specified period of time.
[3]In 1978, there were 203 HMOs in the U.S. serving more than seven million people. HMOs had been certified in 37 states, and 79 were federally qualified. 64 percent of the nation's HMOs were staff or group models (U.S. Department of Health, Education, and Welfare, 1978).

SETTING AND METHODS

Data were gathered from nine HMOs in 1978. They were studied because they include all operational HMOs in a single state and are subject to the same state law and regulations. These HMOs include the three models specified in the federal law. Five of the HMOs are federally qualified, and all are state certified.[4] These HMOs had been operational for one to five years. The number of physicians in staff and group model HMOs ranged from twelve to forty-two, and additional specialists were available for referral in the community. Nearly 600 physicians belonged to IPAs, including both primary care physicians and specialists. The total number of enrollees ranged from approximately 1,000 to 22,000 members. The HMOs are located in urban, suburban, and semi-rural areas.

Sources of data are intensive, open-ended interviews with the HMO executive directors and medical directors, documents provided by the HMOs, and certificates of authority and annual reports filed with the state department of health. Information was collected in three areas in which organizational requirements may affect physician autonomy: reimbursement mechanisms, quality assurance programs, and grievance procedures. These three areas were selected because they are part of the HMO law and, thus, constitute legal requirements for the HMOs; also, these requirements may affect the physician's ability to set the financial value for his or her work, to make individual and independent medical decisions regarding patients, and to control response to patient complaints while being more vulnerable to patient demands.

As noted previously, there are findings which suggest that physician autonomy varies with the degree of bureaucratization of the setting, that organizational bureaucracy includes such characteristics as authority structure and formalization of rules and regulations, and that there are mechanisms by which professionals seek to maximize their autonomy under conditions of organizational constraints. Accordingly, data were gathered concerning who participates in establishing reimbursement, quality assurance, and grievance mechanisms; the extent of codification of the procedures; who has a role in carrying out the procedures; and the enforcement of standards.

---

[4]The state HMO law parallels the federal legislation in requiring a quality review mechanism and a grievance procedure; it does not require that HMO members be on the board of directors of the HMO, as required by federal law.

FINDINGS

The evidence to be presented concerns the implementation of the HMO concept in three areas: (1) physician reimbursement mechanisms, (2) quality assurance programs, and (3) grievance procedures.

Reimbursement Mechanisms

In the staff model, salary negotiation with individual physicians is carried out by the executive director with the whole plan balance sheet in mind, or by the medical director with a budget to allocate among different physicians. In both cases, the budget is subject to review by the board which may include lay or nonprofessional members. Part-time physicians enter the same negotiation process but are reimbursed by capitation. In the group model, salary negotiation occurs among physicians in the group or between a physician and the representative of the medical group. These negotiations are subject to an agreement between the medical group and the HMO about capitation for the group. In both staff and group models, there were reports that negotiations took into account the "market value" differential among specialties. In the IPA model, the medical group contracts with the HMO for payment on a capitation basis; the medical group then reimburses individual physicians on a fee-for-service basis, using a scale based on the "usual and customary" charges of area physicians. Payment is an amount ranging from 80 to 90 percent of physician charges, with the remaining funds constituting a risk pool to cover excess costs to the plan for physicians' services.

Peer Review and Quality Assurance

As guidelines for practice and criteria for review of physician behavior are established, these may be written in the form of a physician handbook or protocols for practice. Five HMOs have written standards that are distributed to physicians. These may encompass administrative matters, including guidelines for record-keeping and rules for scheduling patient appointments, and may specify HMO services and the processes of monitoring how these services are delivered. The protocols also tend to set the tone for medical conduct by stating a general philosophy of medical practice ("...increase the effectiveness and quality of health care provided") or by listing goals of the organization (e.g., high quality care, continuing education for physicians, and patient education).

Standards for medical practice are empirically derived by physicians. The IPAs use standards developed by physician groups in the community (e.g., the county medical society); in the staff and group model plans, the standards are designed by the medical director and/or staff physicians or are derived from the practice patterns of the HMO physicians themselves. As emphasized in several interviews, the standards are intended to be general guidelines which reflect usual patterns of practice and are used to detect deviations from these patterns, not to specify step-by-step procedures for patient care. According to one HMO Certificate of Authority, "the standard does not define good or bad care. It is used to ascertain whether or not a chart or other performance is deviant."

Each HMO has a peer review system in which physicians examine their own records and those of their colleagues in three areas of medical practice: ambulatory care, hospitalization, and referral to specialists. The type of review activity, frequency of review, and person(s) doing the review vary in the different HMOs studied.

Ambulatory review. The initial screening of ambulatory medical records is performed by physicians in all except two of the plans. In all the HMOs, the quality assurance review process is carried out by one or more physicians.[5] Review of charts occurs at regular intervals or at the discretion of the medical director, and frequency of chart review varies from weekly to monthly. Generally, charts to be reviewed are selected at random, by disease category or by outcome. The review processes in these HMOs focus on a variety of items in the charts. In some plans there is a specific list of items to be reviewed, e.g., number of visits, duration of treatment, and prescriptions. As one medical director reported, in looking for deviations from accepted standards and prevailing patterns of practice, the physicians want to "locate weak areas of care."

When a deviation from the standard pattern is found, or if another problem is noted, decisions about what to do vary with the particular issue. In the interviews, executive directors and medical directors reported that physicians were not reprimanded as if performance had been judged inadequate; rather the emphasis is on counseling, educating, and advising physicians. Where the problem is judged to be that of an individual physician, usually the medical director informally brings it to his

---

[5]In two plans, nonphysicians also participate in the quality assurance review process; these include nurses, medical records personnel, and the center director. This participation appears to be an administrative role only, with no input in setting standards.

or her attention. For other problems, the medical director may send a letter discussing the issue to all the physicians rather than singling out a particular physician.

The review process is also used as a basis for revising existing standards of practice within the plan. The review of an individual physician's chart may prompt a review of the records of all physicians in a specific area of practice. If patterns of practice behavior are uncovered that appear to be inappropriate, the group revises the standards. Thus, consensus develops as part of the review process in regard to standards for practice and specific problems which are raised in the record review.

While all the HMOs are required to have ambulatory review procedures, the extent to which these procedures are formalized as rules of the organization varies. As suggested by Aiken and Hage (1966), two aspects are important to consider: the degree of codification of the rules (as in the written physician protocols) and supervision in adherence to these rules (through the quality assurance and review mechanisms). Physicians participate in both of these organizational processes. It is physicians who set the framework within which the ambulatory review process takes place by developing the standards used to judge physician practice, and they are the exclusive participants in seven of the HMOs studied.

Referrals to specialists. Some type of authorization is required for all referrals. In-house referrals must be authorized by the primary care physicians; that is, there are no self-referrals by patients. Referrals to specialists outside the HMO must be countersigned, in most plans by the medical director. This system provides a formal mechanism for review of physician's work in regard to appropriateness of referrals. In one instance, a medical director found that a pediatrician had made an unusual number of referrals to the orthopedic specialist because he felt unsure treating these cases. The pediatrician was sent for a special course in orthopedics, part of the rationale being that it is cheaper to keep simple cases in-house than pay a specialist for referrals.

Referrals to hospitals. A retrospective review of hospitalizations for enrollees exists in all the HMOs. Post-admission review of hospital records and authorization for the admission is made by a nurse or other non-physician who reviews the admission for appropriateness and length of stay according to standards developed by a designated organization of physicians in the community. Subsequent concurrent reviews are conducted at specified intervals to authorize continued hospitalization. This review process is similar to that for physicians in private practice. According to legislation which establishes Professional Standards Review Organizations (PSROs), post-admission reviews of hospitalizations for Medicaid and Medicare patients must be conducted for apropriateness of service and length of stay (Goran, et al., 1975). Some states have enacted legislation to permit third-party payers access to hospital utilization review data, widening the review process for physicians in private practice.

Grievance Procedures

Consistent with federal and state regulations, there are formal grievance procedures developed by each health plan which outline the steps an enrollee may take to register a complaint. A written statement of procedures is provided for the new member; it may be part of the enrollee contract, contained in a member handbook, or available as a separate handout.

In each of the HMOs, the first step is to give the complaint, in written or oral form, to a designated non-physician staff member, such as a member services coordinator, who attempts to resolve the complaint. The next steps in the process vary considerably among the HMOs; complaints are referred to the medical director, the center administrator, the executive director, the appropriate department head, or a review committee which may include physicians and/or board members. Consumer representatives are involved at this interim stage in five of the plans. The HMO Board of Directors has final authority in four of the plans; four have outside arbitration as the final step, and one has a joint committee as the final arbiter. In three HMOs, at least one consumer must be part of the final appeals body. Generally, the medical profession is represented in the grievance process through the medical director. In half of the plans, the medical director has a decision-making role in the formal process; and physicians have a formal role in the grievance structure in three plans.

Although the grievance system establishes a formal mechanism for patient complaints, in their operation, these structures do not appear to have impinged on physician autonomy. In each HMO, the staff has established and maintained a distinction between administrative and medical matters, usually through informal understandings. Very few complaints about individual physicians were reported. Whenever questions regarding medical practice arise, they are referred to the medical director or the physician department chief for review and solution. Most complaints have concerned matters respondents identified as "process" issues, such as the availability of after-hours services, appointment waiting times, and services to which enrollees believe they are entitled. These complaints are considered administrative matters and are referred to the executive director, the center administrator, or the appropriate department head. Interviews indicate that most enrollee grievances are resolved informally, by bringing the complaint to the attention of the physician or other staff person.

DISCUSSION

Given the requirements for reimbursement levels, quality review, and grievance procedures, it might be expected that in settings such as HMOs, the professional norm of autonomy would be in conflict with bureaucratic structures. Data from documents and administrator interviews in nine HMOs indicate that physician autonomy does not appear to be limited by the way in which these structural mechanisms are implemented.

Although forms of reimbursement vary, physicians participate to some extent in how they operate. Individual physician income in staff and group models is set with the active involvement of the physician. Salary and capitation rates are determined through a process of negotiation rather than through use of fixed, predetermined scales. In most cases, the physician negotiates with the medical director rather than the executive director. Rates for physician services in the IPAs are based on prevailing fees in the community. In all HMOs, physicians are involved in setting income levels, permitting the profession to maintain a degree of autonomy in this aspect of practice.

Quality assurance systems represent one form of differentiated role structure (Barber, 1963) which permits physicians to maintain autonomy and limits potential strain between organizational requirements and professional norms. In these HMOs, there is systematized accountability to the medical profession; physicians set the standards for review and carry out the review process. What constitutes autonomy for the profession may not constitute autonomy for the individual physician. Quality assurance procedures subject physicians' work to a review process. Furthermore, the individual physician may be told to alter aspects of medical work which other physicians decide do not meet group standards. The individual physician may respond to this as an intrusion into his practice and an infringement of autonomy, or as an opportunity to improve work through peer discussion.

Through the grievance system in HMOs, physician behavior that might not be subject to challenge by patients in a solo, fee-for-service practice is potentially subject to review. Members have contractual rights with the organization for a set of services, and they can be expected to make demands which may represent a challenge to physicians (Goss, et al., 1977); Freidson, 1975). It is the grievance procedure which provides a vehicle for patient complaints. In these HMOs, few complaints have been raised about individual physicians. Those grievances that have been voiced were settled informally, after referral to the medical director, without going beyond this first step in the grievance procedure. It seems that in the daily routines of the HMOs, physician autonomy has not been challenged by members.

Comparing these structural features among the three types of HMOs, there is variation (1) in the relationship of professionals to the organization, and (2) in the degree of formalization of procedures and the formal role for different organizational participants. As Hall (1968) and Engel (1969) have shown, such differences, as components of bureaucratization, may be related to levels of autonomy.

Considering the relationship of professionals to the organization,[6] the IPA is distinguished from staff and group models in several respects. IPA physicians may not practice in a group setting; only a portion of their patients are HMO enrollees; they are paid on the usual fee-for-service basis; and as HMO physicians they are members of a physicians' group which contracts with the HMO for the provision of member services. This group has a formal relationship to the plan, and mutual obligations between the HMO and the physician members are detailed. Compared to physicians in staff and group models, the IPA physicians are more similar to the "ideal type" physician in terms of practice setting and reimbursement arrangement. They are similar to physicians in the group model in having a formal contractual relation with the HMO for the provision of member services as part of a physician group.

There is evidence of a continuum of organizational types based on the dimension of degree of formalization of procedures and rules for quality assurance and member grievance. The IPA models appear to be the most formalized and structured; the group model is a mixed type; and the staff model is the least formalized. In the IPA models, there are written proctocols for practice and a medical group review committee for quality assurance. The member grievance system includes a formal role for the medical director and for physicians, and consumers are included in the final appeals procedure within the

---

[6]In all the HMOs, a physician serves in the administrative role of medical director; this position provides a differentiated authority structure (Barber, 1963), a professional authority structure to which the physicians are subject.

plan. While some of the staff model HMOs have written protocols for practice and a formal role for the medical director in the grievance system, none has a formal role for physicians, and none requires that consumers be part of the final appeals body within the plan. The group model HMOs are divided, paralleling the structures in either the IPA or staff models.

From the data on structure in these HMOs, it appears that the IPA model offers greater opportunity for maintaining autonomy of the profession as a whole than do other models. In one case, the local PSRO is closely associated with the medical group and sets the review standards for the IPA, thus consolidating the position of the profession. Because the IPAs appear to be more formalized and more structured than the other models, with physicians establishing and implementing the structure, it is likely that IPA physicians are less subject to controls from outside the profession.

The staff models in this study tend to operate on a more informal basis with fewer prescribed situations in which physicians participate. Perhaps because the physicians practice in a central location, commuication and observability may facilitate the development of informal norms which support individual physician autonomy. Physicians in staff and group models, while subject to the structural requirements of the HMO, appear to have the opportunity to participate in implementing these requirements, and in so doing to negotiate their relationship to the organization, thus maintaining autonomy. Another possibility is that individual professionals may vary in their conformity to professional and bureaucratic norms; for example, the HMO staff physicians may value organizational requirements set forth to promote patient interests and feel that these do not limit autonomy with regard to practice.

IMPLICATIONS AND CONCLUSIONS

The bureaucratic structure of HMOs provides a setting in which professional norms may be challenged. From the available evidence, it appears that physician autonomy may not be diminished by the structural mechanisms for physician reimbursement, quality assurance, and member grievances. Rather, the medical profession, as well as individual physicians, are involved in defining and implementing these mechanisms. These requirements were established by the HMO legislation as part of an attempt to rationalize the health care system and make it more responsive to consumers by providing accessible high quality care at a reasonable cost, and in so doing to focus on prevention of illness and maintenance of health.

The data on HMO organizational characteristics reported in this paper suggest several implications for these broad goals. The process of negotiating their own income is one way that physicians may become more aware of the financial concerns of the HMO, and they may take these into account in decision-making about individual treatments. The different hospitalization rates among staff, group, and IPA models (U.S. Department of Health, Education, and Welfare, 1978) may to some degree reflect differential physician participation in financial issues. On the other hand, physician pressures for higher reimbursement may lead to increased costs for the HMO.

To the extent that practice standards become codified as part of quality assurance requirements, there may be increased rationalization of medical knowledge. In the HMOs studied, there were variations in the extent of codification and the rules for enforcement. Physicians maintained autonomy in both establishing and carrying out the quality assurance programs, and no nonphysicians or consumers participated in a meaningful way in assuring quality of care. These observations suggest that while medical knowledge may become more rationalized and physician accountability more systematized, medical care remains the responsibility of physicians and the medical profession. It has been suggested that in the face of policies intended to alter practice patterns, physicians may maintain dominance while becoming more routinely accountable (Goss, et al., 1977).

The grievance process in HMOs consists of detailed procedures which HMO members are informed about and encouraged to use. This complaint structure is an entry point for the consumers of health services to express objections when they are dissatisfied with organizational practices and the way services are provided. Yet, in these HMOs, members have few complaints and those that are voiced are easily resolved. Whether HMO members are more satisfied consumers cannot be judged from these data. It may be that HMOs are more responsive to consumer interests, or that given a structured opportunity to register specific complaints, consumers are reluctant to do so and need more time to become familiar with this mechanism.

The more rapid rate of growth of IPA models (U.S. Department of Health, Education, and Welfare, 1978:10) suggests that physicians may be seeking ways to maintain autonomy of the medical profession in an increasingly bureaucratic environment. This model allows for decentralized practice sites and traditional practice arrangements (either solo or group practice) while changing the method of financing to a prepayment mechanism. It is not clear whether this model will substantially lower costs and improve quality as well as physician accountability to the public.

Generalizations from these data are limited by the number of HMOs and the geographic area of the country in which they are located. It is suggested that through physician participation in organizational mechanisms, the potential for clash between bureaucratic requirements and the professional norm of autonomy may be reduced. There is differential participation by physicians in nego-tiating salary and reimbursement, as well as in the establishment and operation of quality assurance mecha-nisms and member grievance procedures. These variations suggest that individual physician participation in these mechanisms will be related to perceptions of autonomy, and that physician responses will vary in the different HMO models. To study these issues, evidence is needed about physicians' involvement in organizational decision-making and their perceptions of autonomy under varying organizational conditions.

REFERENCES

Aiken, Michael and Jerald Hage
    1966   "Organizational Alienation: A Comparative
            Analysis." American Sociological Review 31
            (August):497-507.
Barber, Bernard
    1963   "Some Problems in the Sociology of the
            Professions." Daedalus 92 (Fall):669-688.
Blau, Peter M. and W. Richard Scott
    1961   Formal Organizations. San Francisco:
            Chandler Publishing Company.
Bucher, Rue and Anselm Strauss
    1961   "Professions in Process." American Journal
            of Sociology 66 (January):325-334.
Child, John and Janet Schriescheim
    1978   "Changes in the Social Position of Profes-
            sional Occupations." Paper presented at the
            American Sociological Association Annual
            Meeting, San Francisco, September.
Ellwood, Paul M., Jr., Nancy N. Anderson, James E.
            Billings, Rick J. Carlson, Earl J. Hoagberg,
            and Walter McClure
    1971   "Health Maintenance Strategy." Medical Care
            9 (May-June):291-298.
Engel, Gloria V.
    1969   "The Effect of Bureaucracy on the Profes-
            sional Autonomy of the Physician." Journal
            of Health and Social Behavior 10 (March):
            30-41.
Etzioni, Amitai
    1961   A Comparative Analysis of Complex Organiza-
            tions. New York: The Free Press.
Freidson, Eliot
    1970   Profession of Medicine: A Study in the
            Sociology of Applied Knowledge. New York:
            Dodd, Mead.

1975   Doctoring Together. New York: Elsevier Press.
Goran, Michael J., James S. Roberts, Meg A. Kellogg,
        Jonathan Fielding, and William Jessee
    1975   "The PSRO Hospital Review System." Medical
                Care 13 (April):1-33 Supplement.
Goss, Mary E.W.
    1961   "Influence and Authority Among Physicians in
                an   Out-Patient   Clinic."   American
                Sociological Review 26 (February):29-50.
Goss, Mary E.W., Roger M. Battistella, John Colombotos,
        Eliot Freidson, and Donald C. Riedel
    1977   "Social Organization and Control in Medical
                Work: A Call for Research." Medical Care 15
                (May):1-10.
Hall, Richard H.
    1968   "Professionalization and Bureaucratization."
                American Sociological Review 33 (February):
                92-104.
Haug, Marie R.
    1976   "The Erosion of Professional Authority: A
                Cross-Cultural Inquiry in the Case of the
                Physician." Milbank Memorial Fund Quarterly
                (Winter):83-106.
Larson, Magali Sarfatti
    1977   The Rise of Professionalism: A Sociological
                Analysis.   Berkeley: University   of
                California Press.
Litwak, Eugene
    1961   "Models   of   Bureaucracy   Which   Permit
                Conflict." American Journal of Sociology 67
                (September): 177-184.
Madison, Donald L., Hugh H. Tilson, and Thomas R. Konrad
    1977   "Physician   Recruitment,   Retention,   and
                Satisfaction in Medical Practice Organiza-
                tions."   Health Services Research Center,
                Univeristy of North Carolina at Chapel Hill,
                December.
Nathanson, Constance and Marshall H. Becker
    1972   "Control   Structure   and   Conflict   in
                Outpatient Clinics."   Journal of Health and
                Social Behavior 13 (September):251-262.
Roth, Julius
    1974   "Professionalism: The Sociologist's Decoy."
                Sociology   of   Work   and   Occupations   1
                (February):6-23.
Scott, W. Richard
    1966   "Professionals in Bureaucracies: Areas of
                Conflict." Pp. 265-275 in
                Professionalization. Howard M. Vollmer and
                Donald L. Mills, Editors. Englewood Cliffs,
                New   Jersey: Prentice   Hall,   Inc.

44

Thompson, Victor
    1961   Modern Organizations. New York: Alfred A
            Knopf.
U.S. Department of Health, Education, and Welfare
    1977   Health Maintenance Organizations, Interim
            Regulations. Federal Register. Wednesday,
            June 8, Part II.
U.S. Department of Health, Education, and Welfare
    1978   National HMO Census of Prepaid Plans 1978.
            Public Health Service.   Office of Health
            Maintenance Organizations.

4
The Paradoxes of Health Planning

Bonnie Morel Edington
Health Planning Services, New Jersey Department of Health

The National Health Planning Act of 1974 designated 200 Health Systems Agencies (HSAs) nationally and a State Health Planning and Development Agency in each state. Components of the law are analyzed to illustrate its ambiguities and contradictions. The components analyzed are: the findings which led to the passage of the law; the law's purpose; the ten national health priorities; the National Guidelines for Health Planning; the purposes of the HSAs and the data they are to assemble and analyze. The major contradiction is that agencies designated to focus on cost containment in health care are expected to make health care services more accessible and acceptable, and improve their quality. These agencies are also expected to improve the health of the population, including ill health attributable to environmental factors.

Social policy regarding prevention is discussed, particularly the current trend toward blaming the victim. Contradictions and ironies in planning for cost containment are also pointed out: patients are blamed for utilization that is provider-induced; there is no constiuency for cost containment; consumers (i.e., purchasers) with the greatest potential clout are large employers and organized labor, but such labor-management coalitions are just beginning to be developed; Certificates of Need require no proof of need; and current anti-regulation fervor may not distinguish state health planning regulations for cost containment, such as those adopted in New Jersey, from the cost-generating regulations of most government agencies.

The National Health Planning and Resources Development Act of 1974 designated a State Health Planning and Development Agency in each state, and 200 local Health Systems Agencies (HSAs) to plan for discrete areas that blanketed the country. The law also established a Statewide Health Coordinating Council whose members are appointed by the Governor, 60 percent of these appointees being nominated by the HSA, and at least half being non-providers of health care. Each HSA produces a plan, and the Council, staffed by the state planning agency, compiles these into a State Health Plan.

The law has been called one of the most complex pieces of modern legislation and it give HSAs conflicting and contradictory mandates. In its "Findings and Purpose" section it states first that "equal access to quality health care at a reasonable cost is a priority of the Federal Government," then goes on to say that: The "massive infusion of Federal funds into the existing health care system has contributed to inflationary increases in the cost of health care and failed to produce an adequate supply or distribution of health resources," which has inhibited equal access; there are inadequate incentives for the use of appropriate alternatives to inpaient care; and "large segments of the public are lacking in basic knowledge regarding proper personal health care and methods for effective use of available health services."

There is a section in the law on the ten national health priorities:

1. provision of primary care services for the medically underserved;
2. coordination and consolidation of hospital services;
3. development of group practices and health maintenance organization (HMOs);
4. increased use of physician assistants;
5. coordination and consolidation of hospital support services;
6. improvement in the quality of health services;
7. geographic integration of levels of care;
8. prevention of disease;
9. improvement of hospital management procedures; and
10. effective health education for the public.

There is also a section on national guidelines for health planning, which states that within eighteen months of the passage of the law, guidelines were to be issued concerning national health planning policy. The guidelines were to be of two types: standards for the appropriate supply, distribution, and organization of health resources; and a statement of national health planning goals expressed in quantitative terms, the goals to be developed after considering the national health priorities. The law was signed January 4, 1975, and, as of September, 1979, only one document with eleven standards had appeared in final form, March 28, 1978, fifteen months behind schedule.

These National Health Planning Guidelines specified: maximum numbers of beds in ratio to population for the three major types of hospital services -- general medical-surgical, obstetric, and pediatric; minimum occupancy levels in those services; and minimum numbers of specialized procedures (e.g., obstetrical deliveries, open heart surgery, and CAT scans) to be done at a single site.

The standards for maximum numbers of beds are intended to prevent resource duplication and thereby restrain costs. The standards regarding minimum numbers of procedures are intended not only to prevent duplication and restrain costs, but also to encourage consolidation of services so that adequate utilization, quality of care and, to some degree, health can be improved. The standards were based on well-established research findings and recommendations by the appropriate medical professional organizations. Data indicate that as the numbers of procedures increase, including routine obstetrical procedures, the mortality rate among patients declines, since the medical team gains proficiency.

The law states that HSAs are to do their planning for seven purposes:

1. to improve health;
2. to increase the accessibility of health services;
3. to increase the acceptability of health services;
4. to increase the continuity of health services;
5. to increase the quality of health services;
6. to restrain costs; and
7. to prevent unnecessary duplication of services.

The law then states that the HSAs are to "assemble" and analyze data on the health of the population, the health care delivery system, the effect the health care delivery system has on the health of the population, and the environmental and occupational exposure factors affecting the health of the population. But it also states they are not to collect data; they are to use existing data.

The law instructs the HSAs to consider the national priorities, the national guidelines, and the pre-existing data in preparing their plan, which is to "describe a healthful environment and health system which, when developed, will assure that quality services... (are) available and accessible in a manner which assures continuity of care, at reasonable cost, for all residents of the area... ."

The chart 4.1 is an analysis of the degree of overlap between and among: the factors that surfaced in the findings that led to the law; the national health priorities; the HSAs' purposes as stated in the law; the type of data HSAs are supposed to assemble and analyze;

and the National Health Planning Guidelines. The diagram illustrates a major ambiguity in the law - are planners being paid primarily to control costs or to improve health?

As can be seen in the first column of the diagram, none of the findings that led to the law were directly related to the health of the population. Only the need for health education of the public seems to reflect it, and even that is oblique since the focus seemed to be more on health education to reduce over utilization of services. The findings did not cite any diseases or health conditions as problematic, nor did it imply that health services were so lacking, or so poor in quality, that a negative impact on the health of the population had resulted.

As the bottom line of the second column shows, only three of the national health priorities can be construed as remotely aimed at health improvement - prevention, health education, and quality of services, and even so, "quality" can mean a great many things other than clearly improved outcome in health status. The most notable thing in the second column is the fact that seven of the ten national health priorities are related to cost containment.

Yet, as the third column shows, the HSAs are told their primary purpose is to improve health; their secondary purpose is to make health sevices even more ubiquitous, attractive, overutilized, comprehensive and expensive, i.e.., "to increase accessibility, acceptability, continuity and quality" of services. And then they are told to restrain costs and prevent duplication.

Their instructions regarding data underscore the paradox. These local agencies, in areas with relatively small populations, are to answer questions that have been addressed by numerous studies at the National Institutes of Health and the National Center for Health Services Research, that is, they are to analyze the "environmental and occupational exposure factors affecting the health of the population" and "the effect the health care delivery system has on the health of the population, without collecting any data (df. Klarman, 1978). The existing health data available to them on local residents consists mainly of vital statistics, reportable diseases that have almost no connection to the hospital services for which they must plan, and mortality data that tells little of incidence, prevalence or etiology of the chronic diseases related to environment and occupation. Data available to them from the National Center for Health Statistics are based on national samples so small that they cannot be disaggregated for local areas, nor even for states.

On October 4, 1979, the Health Planning Law was amended to authorize the Secretary of HEW to: "collect data to determine whether the health care delivery

49

TABLE 4.1

Findings were related to	National Health Priorities	HSA Purposes	HSA Data
Inaccessibility	1.Primary care for medically underserved 4.Increased use of physician assistants	2.Increasing accessibility	
INFLATIONARY COSTS*	2.COORDIN./CONSOLID. OF HOSP. SERVICES 3.Development of group practices/HMOs 4.Increased use of physician assistants 5.Coordin./consolid. of support services 7.Geog. integration of levels of care 8.Prevention 9.Improvement of hosp. mgt. procedures	6.RESTRAINING COSTS	
MALDISTRIBUTION OF RESOURCES	1.Primary care for medically underserved 2.COORDIN./CONSOLID. OF HOSP. SERVICES 4.Increased use of physician assistants 7.Geog. integration of levels of care	7.PREVENTING RESOURCE DUPLICATION 4.Increasing continuity of care	
Need for incentives for alternatives to inpatient care	3.Development of group practices/HMOs 8.Prevention		
Need for health education of public	8.Prevention 10.Effective health educ. of publlic	1.Improving health	
	6.IMPROVEMENT IN QUALITY OF SERVICES	1.IMPROVING HEALTH 3.Increasing acceptability 5.Increasing quality	

Health system and its utilization

Health status

Environmental and occupa-tional exposure

Health status

systems meet or are changing to meet" the goals included
in the plans of HSAs and state planning agencies; "prescribe the manner in which such data shall be assembled
and reported"; and analyze the data. The amendments also
added seven national health priorities, which seem to
bear the following relationship to the findings that led
to the original law, the other national health priorities, and the HSAs' purposes:

TABLE 4.2

Findings that led to original law	New (additional) National Health Priorities	HSA Purposes
Inflationary costs	11. Energy conservation in health facilities	6. Restraining costs
Inflationary costs and maldistribution	12. Identification and discontinuance of duplicative or unneeded services and facilities	6. Restraining costs 7. Preventing resource duplication
Inflationary costs; maldistribution; need for health education of public	13. Adoption of policies which will: contain rapidly rising costs; promote efficiency; insure more appropriate use of services	6. Restraining costs 7. Preventing resource duplication
Need for incentives for alternatives to inpatient care	14. Elimination of inappropriate placement in institutions of persons with mental health problems, and improvement of the quality of care in mental health institutions.	3. Increasing acceptability 5. Increasing quality
Inaccessibility; mal-distribution; need for incentives for alternatives to inpatient care	15. Increased accessibility of outpatient alternatives for mental health services	2. Increasing accessibility 3. Increasing acceptability
	16. Promotion of services provided "in a manner cognizant of emotional and psychological components of prevention, treatment and maintenance of health"	3. Increasing acceptability 5. Increasing quality
Inflationary costs and inaccessibility	17. Strengthening of competition in health industry where it 'advances the purposes of quality assurance, cost effectiveness, and access"	2. Increasing accessibility 5. Increasing quality 6. Restraining costs

Priorities 12 and 13 are an expansion of priority 2,
coordination and consolidation of hospital services;
priorities 14, 15, 16, and 17 are related to priority 6,
improvement in quality. Although cost containment is
implied in priorities 11, 12, 13, and 17, this is offset
by the cost-generating implications of 14, 15, 16, and 17
-- accessibility, acceptability and quality. It is also
noteworthy that priorities 14, 15, and 16 are the only
ones that address a particular health status condition
-- mental health. And not only do the new priorities
give further evidence of what has been called the
"schizophrenia of the feds" regarding health status and

costs, but they introduce a new paradox unrelated to health status -- the "strengthening of competition" while consolidating services and preventing resource duplication.

HEALTH STATUS AND PUBLIC POLICY -- BLAMING THE VICTIM

Economic and social class factors related to lifestyle, nutrition, environment and occupation are the major predictors of health status. A relatively small proportion of the variance in health status is attributable to the medical care system in this country (cf. Fuchs, 1974; Knowles, 1977; Leveson, 1979; McKinlay and McKinlay, 1977; Rice, 1976). This fact has led to a new form of blaming the victim (cf. Crawford, 1977). Proponents of the new "holistic health" and "wellness" ideologies are sometimes reminiscent of fundamentalist preachers in suggesting that those who become ill must not have been living right. Insurance companies publish full-page ads in national magazines explaining why health care costs are skyrocketing. These depict people sitting in their living rooms watching television and snacking, in the park playing ball and drinking beer with paunchy friends on weekends, and working at their desks after 11 p.m. These appear to be among the things John Knowles, M.D., a prominent figure in health policy-making until his recent death (at age 52, of cancer) has described on national television and in a number of mass publications as the "personal misbehavior" responsible for health problems.

Making people feel responsible for their own behavior is good psychology; it helps to bring about the desired results. But it is poor policy-making and irresponsible governing to implement no incentive or disincentive system to elicit that desired behavior. It can reasonably be argued that those in government who hold the public responsible are, themselves, abrogating responsibility in public service (cf. Etzioni, 1977).

To address the health status problems related to consumer lifestyle, policy-makers must find ways to limit the availability and accessibility of the products in question (e.g., tobacco, alcohol, non-nutritious foods), making them just difficult enough to obtain to somewhat reduce the demand, which would then reduce the supply. The related industries must then be encouraged and assisted in diverting to more socially beneficial products. The less beneficial must again be made slightly more unavailable, and so on. There must be a fine tuning and gradual adjustment throughout the process, to assure that it is always short of coercion and diminishing returns in the social system. There would appear to be a great deal of latitude for public policy between the one extreme of making something illegal, which can be disruptive to the economic system and lead to a black market, and the other extreme of letting industry dictate public policy. There has been a tendency toward the latter extreme in this country.

Recent studies have shown that the tobacco industry has benefitted even from ostensibly anti-smoking governmental actions. When broadcasters were prohibited from advertising cigarettes they were also freed of the obligation to broadcast anti-smoking messages, and smoking increased; the ban on broadcast advertising kept new cigarette firms out and permitted the six major firms to control over 99 percent of the market (cf. Doron, 1979). Furthermore, policy that protects the tobacco industry on the grounds that numerous jobs are involved and the economy of large regions that would otherwise be in poverty, and simultaneously castigates the smokers whose purchases assure that those people are fed, is policy without credibility (cf. Markle and Troyer, 1979).

This chapter will not address the deficiencies of federal policy in regard to health status problems connected to environmental, industrial, and occupational factors. Those may well be the major health status problems, but health planning agencies cannot really be expected to deal with them. The Congressional Record of July 7, 1978, shows that Congress is attempting to provide HSAs with a "clearer delineation of intended scope" and wished to direct them away from "amorphous areas" such as "air quality," but some HSAs are objecting to this directive (cf. Higgins and Philips, 1979). They may wish to deal with these issues in general terms, but the chances that HSAs will point fingers at major industries responsible for health problems is minimal, given the fact that these politically vulnerable agencies are reluctant even to name the superfluous hospitals that need to close (Huppert et al., 1979).

HEALTH CARE OVERUTILIZATION - BLAMING THE VICTIM

Much of the literature implies the public is replete with hypochondriacs, overutilizers and abusers of the health care system. In reality, many of the annual check-ups, Pap smears, and so on, that are now deemed inappropriate for low-risk persons, were check-ups everyone was urged to get in the recent past. People who were compliant are now told they abused the system. The patient only initiates contact with the threshhold of the health care system and, after that, the drugs, the return visits, the hospital admission, the surgery, are all at the behest of the physician gatekeeper (cf. Fuchs, 1974; Ginzberg, 1978; Klarman, 1978; Stone, 1979).

People are now told they should get second opinions before undergoing any surgery, since research has shown that will reduce the amount of unnecessary surgery. When the second opinion differs from the first, a tie-breaking third must be sought. But getting a second or third opinion increases the number of initial visits to a doctor's office (the second and third doctor), so that statistic may increase and the so-called "worried well" again faulted for overutilization.

COST CONTAINMENT AND HEALTH PLANNING

Over the last ten years, the cost of hospital care has risen more than twice as fast as the total cost of living (cf. U.X. DHEW, 1978). As Sally Berger (1978), Chairman of the National Council on Health Planning and Development, has stated, health planners need a policy that articulates their mission: "To contain costs without detriment to health." Foisting health status problems onto health planning agencies funded at less than 50 cents per capita impedes planners' ability to focus effectively on problems in the health care system related to cost containment. Health care providers struggling for individual economic survival, prestige and prosperity in an industry that needs to retrench would not be averse to having planning agencies diverted from cost containment into finding more patients for their services, particularly in they are patients who can be blamed for their own illnesses and for any ineffectiveness of treatment.

Virtually all attempts to resolve problems of health care financial inaccessibility have resulted in greater benefits to providers than to consumers. Medicare and Medicaid had unintended and unanticipated incentives to provider-induced overutilization that have now struck legitimate fear into the hearts of advocates of national health insurance (cf. Newhose et al., 1977). Policy-makers have learned that programs extending even parsimonious payment for what were intended to be the clearest cut cases of need, have inevitably offered undue and unforseen incentives to providers of care. "Rationing of health care," a phrase now being used by policy-makers, may already be occurring. Holding the line on government spending for health care, while the cost of health services steadily increases, means that fewer persons received services for those dollars being held constant.

Yet there is no real constituency for cost containment. In 1977, 70 percent of personal health care expenditures, and 94 percent of hospital expenditures, were covered by third-party insurers. Government-supported programs paid 40 percent of all personal health care, and 55 percent of hospital care (cf. U.S. DHEW, 1978). These costs are passed on to the individual taxpayer and the payer of insurance premiums, but the taxpayer is seldom aware of how much of his or her taxes are earmarked for health care, and the impact on individual premium payers has been greatly mitigated by the fact that employers have been paying an ever-increasing proportion of these premiums. It is a basic social fact that spreading any cost burden more evenly reduces the likelihood that anyone will be affected enough to care about the cost (cf. Hiatt, 1975).

The National Health Planning Law states that the majority of members of the HSA's governing body shall be consumers of health care who are not providers, the intent being to prevent provider domination of health planning. "Major purchasers of health care" are mentioned last in a list of consumer types, and insurers, even though they clearly have a vested interest in containing costs, are specifically deemed "providers." It has not been made sufficiently clear that the "consumer" is meant to be someone who has as strong an interest in and knowledge about restraining the health care system as providers of health care have interest in and knowledge about expanding it. And this consumer representative should have some political clout equal to that of the health providers. Such consumers may be the employers who pay large premiums for group insurance as part of the fringe benefits offered to employees. Individual premium payers do not have enough of a stake in cost containment to warrant committing themselves to it, they cannot sit on health planning boards and councils on company time as representatives of large employers can, and they cannot provide the countervailing balance to provider interests that industry can.

Organized labor is coming to realize that its members are not eager to gain greater health benefits at the cost of net loss in real earnings (cf. Council on Wage and Price Stability, 1976). Labor organizations are now specified as "major purchasers" of health care in new amendments to the health planning law. Nationwide the number of health sector jobs to be lost if cost-containment measures are taken is not likely to be prohibitive, although the potential loss of jobs due to hospital closure looms exceptionally large in New York City politically and is a highly publicized and volatile issue there.

Labor-management coalitions are forming to take a more active role in health care cost-containment and may prove to be a potent force (cf. Goldbeck, 1978).

IMPLEMENTATION OF PLANS

The only legally effective tool that HSAs have to implement cost containment plans is the Certificate of Need (CN). State laws specify that health facilities wishing to expand their buildings or services must apply for a CN. HSAs tend to devote one-quarter to one-half of their staff resources to reviewing these applications and they recommend approval or disapproval to the Statewide Health Coordinating Council which, in turn, makes a recommendation to the state agency which is legally authorized to grant the CN. Federal monies are withheld from facilities violating state CN laws.

HSAs tend to recommend approval, but rarely because of "need," more commonly because any new service or building is a clear-cut addition to that community, whether or not it is needed, or adequately or appropriately utilized. It provides jobs, if nothing else. If it is disapproved for reasons of cost containment, the money saved is not money the community gets to spend on some other, more necessary service in its own area exclusively; the savings are spread across the country. So the indisputable logic is, "If we put it here, whatever the gain in service, it's totally our gain and the cost is only fractionally ours. If we keep it out, the savings are fractionally ours, and the service gain is zero to everyone."

This logic and the power of individual providers has meant that unless there are competing CN applications, planners reviewing these applications rarely have to justify approval but are nearly always forced to justify denial. The burden of proof is not on the applicant and "Certificate of Need" has proved to be a misnomer; it might more accurately be termed a "Certificate of Acquiescence."

CN laws are only designed to limit or control growth and, even so, most studies indicate they have had little success (cf. Ginzberg, 1978; Klarman, 1976 and 1978; Wendling, 1978). CN applications must be initiated by providers, and the planners' role is reactive. CN does not provide an implementation tool for planning initiatives directed at contraction of the health care industry - consolidation and closure of unnecessary facilities and services. The potential tools for contraction are not in the hands of HSAs, but rest with state agencies, which license health facilities, make the ultimate CN decisions (sometimes using HSA staff analyses that were ignored by provider-influenced HSA boards), set the reimbursement rates that third-party payers are allowed to pay hospitals, and pass regionalization regulations (cf. Altman, 1978). State rate-setting is relatively new, exists in only a few states, and is usually limited to Medicaid and/or Blue Cross reimbursement. However, New Jersey has a new law which will permit the state planning agency to set rates for all third-party payers.

The National Guidelines for Health Planning referred to earlier are intended to be used to effect contraction, consolidation and closure. They were late and limited because they had to run the gauntlet. As sound, well-documented and well-established as these standards were, the provider hue and cry resounded throughout the nation.

In seventy-seven days of public comment 55,000 communications were received and five public hearings were held. Some of the standards had to be lowered, and federal planners may be reluctant to undergo another such barrage in the foreseeable future. But state and HSA planners need many more such criteria and standards in order to function effectively. In New Jersey state planners had written state regionalization regulations and plans around most of the above standards and criteria a year before the federal guidelines appeared. Other states may have to develop and pass regulations with only covert support from federal agencies.

The last paradox of health planning is that the current antitaxation/anti-government movement is not likely to distinguish between govermental units which provide services and pass regulations which increase costs, and those agencies which are designed to reduce unnecessary services and restrain costs through regulation.

SUMMARY

A health care cornucopia led to runaway inflation in costs. The National Health Planning Law was originally intended to control and curtail the proliferation of health services, distributing them more rationally and economically. But the law led to the establishment of health planning agencies that are expected to

1. grapple with the causes of disease in small areas for which data do not exist and cannot be collected;
2. improve health status by planning for services which do not significantly affect the health status of a population;
3. improve the services while reducing their cost; and
4. keep the services to a minimum by persuading local power-wielders that they should be altruistic, foregoing services in their own area so that taxpayers in 199 other areas of the country can benefit.

Meanwhile, real health status problems are being attributed to bad habits and immorality of individuals using products that are manufactured, distributed and widely advertised under an industry-protective public policy.

If health planning agencies are to justify their existence they must be allowed to focus on restraining, converting, consolidating and closing excess health services. They must develop a constituency for cost containment. They must have planning criteria and standards that become legally binding through state and federal legislation.

REFERENCES

Altman, Drew
  1978   "The Politics of Health Care Regulation:
            The care of the National Health Planning and
            Resources Development Act." Journal of
            Health Politics, Policy and Law, 2:560-580.
Berger, Sally
  1978   "Health Planning for Georgia -- Looking Ahead
            To The '80s." Speech given at Callaway
            Gardens, Pine Mountain, Ga., September 22.
Council on Wage and Price Stability, Executive Office of
            the President
  1976   The Complex Puzzle of Rising Health Care
            Costs: Can the Private Sector Fit It
            Together?   Washington,   D.C.:   U.S.
            Government Printing Office.
Crawford, R.
  1977   "You Are Dangerous to Your Health: The
            Ideology and Politics of Victim Blaming."
            International Journal of Health Services,
            7:663-680.
Doron, Gideon
  1979   "Administrative Regulation of an Industry:
            The Cigarette Case." Public Administration
            Review, 39:163-170.
Etzioni, Amitai
  1977   "Health As A Social Priority." In Arthur
            Levin (ed.), Health Services: The Local
            Perspecitve.   New York: Academy of
            Political Science.
Fuchs, Victor R.
  1974   Who Shall Live?   Health, Economics and
            Social Choice. New York: Basic Books.
Ginzberg, Eli
  1978   "Health Reform: The Outlook For The 1980s."
            Inquiry 15:311-326.
Goldbeck, Willis B.
  1978   A Business Perspective on Industry and
            Health Care. New York: Springer.
Hiatt, H. H.
  1975   "Protecting The Medical Commons: Who Is
            Responsible?" New England Journal of
            Medicine. 293:235-241.
Higgins, Charles Wayne and Bill U. Philips
  1979   "Taking 'Health' Out of Health Planning."
            Health Values-Achieving High Level Wellness.
            3:209-211.
Huppert, Michael, Robert Bradbury and Robert Higgins
  1979   "Institution Specificity In Acute Care Plan-
            ning -- The Central Massachusetts experi-
            ence." Paper presented at the American
            Public Health Association meeting, New York.

58

Klarman, Herbert E.
    1976   "National Policies and Local Planning for
            Health Services."   Milbank Memorial Fund
            Quarterly/Health and Society. 54:1-28.
    1978   "Health Planning: Progress, Prospects, and
            Issues." Milbank Memorial Fund Quarterly/
            Health and Society. 56:78-112.
Knowles, John, editor
    1977   Doing Better and Feeling Worse: Health in
            the United States. New York: Norton.
Leveson, Irving
    1979   "Some Policy Implications of the Relation-
            ship Between Health Services and Health."
            Inquiry. 16:9-21.
McKinlay, John B. and Sonja M. McKinlay
    1977   "The Questionable Contribution of Medical
            Measures to the Decline of Mortality in the
            United States in the Twentieth Century."
            Milbank Memorial Fund Quarterly/Health and
            Society. 55:405-428.
Markle, Gerald E. and Ronald J. Troyer
    1979   "Smoke Gets in Your Eyes: Cigarette Smoking
            as Deviant Behavior."   Social Problems.
            26:611-625.
Newhouse, Joseph P., Charles E. Phelps and William B.
            Schwartz
    1977   "Policy Options and the Impact of National
            Health Insurance." In Robert H. Haveman and
            Julius Margolis (eds.), Public Expenditure
            and Policy Analysis, 2nd ed. Chicago: Rand
            MaNally.
Rice, Dorothy P.
    1979   "The American Medical Economy: Problems and
            Perspectives." Journal of Health Politics,
            Policy and Law 1:151-172.
Stone, Deborah A.
    1979   "Physicians as Gatekeepers: Illness Cer-
            tification as a Rationing Device."   Public
            Policy 27:227-254.
U.S. Department of Health, Education, and Welfare
    1978   Health: United States 1978. Hyattsville,
            Md.: National Center for Health Statistics
            and National Center for Health Services
            Research.
Wendling, Wayne
    1978   "A   Reexamination   of   the   Impact   of
            Certificate-of-Need Laws."   In Jack L.
            Werner and Jacqueline R. Leopold (eds.),
            Socioeconomic Issues of Health 1978.
            Monroe, Wisc.: American Medical Association.

5

Mission Neighborhood Health Center: A Case Study of the Department of Health, Education and Welfare as a Counterinsurgency Agency

*Thomas S. Bodenheimer
and Marlene Dixon*
Institute for the Study of Labor and Economic Crisis

In the 1960s, working class communities all over the country, particularly minority inner city neighborhoods, exploded in violent anger. The federal government responded with a pacification or cooling-out program: the War on Poverty. The War on Poverty provided federal funds to bring a few programs into the community, to create a few jobs, and to buy off working class leaders who were a threat to those in power. In the course of this program of counterinsurgency, the War on Poverty took over a slogan of the 1960s, "community control," and turned it into its opposite; rather than control by the community, "community control" came to mean control over the working class majority of the community.

One of the War on Poverty's important programs was the neighborhood health center program to provide ambulatory health care to low income people. This program, initially slated to reach 25 million people through 1,000 health centers, was scaled down to 125 centers serving only 1.5 million people. The standard view of the neighborhood health center program holds that its aims were

1. to bring high quality health care to people previously denied such care,
2. to provide employment opportunities and training

The Institute for the Study of Labor and Economic Crisis was requested by Mission Neighborhood Health Center patients to assist in their fight for democratic elections and decent health care. This paper reflects the Institute's understanding gained through active participation in this struggle.

This article originally appeared in Health Care in Crisis, Essays on Health Services Under Capitalism, Marlene Dixon and Thomas Bodenheimer, M.D., editors (Synthesis Publications, P.O. Box 40099, San Francisco, CA 94140), 1980.

60

          to neighborhood residents, and
3. to allow community members to participate in the governance of health centers (Davis and Schoen, 1978).

A more realistic view sees the neighborhood health center program as a means to control, rather than to assist, minority working class populations. This paper takes the example of one neighborhood health center, Mission Neighborhood Health Center in San Francisco, to show how federal counterinsurgency works in the 1970s and to expose the class character of "community control."

THE EXPLOITATION OF PATIENTS AT MISSION NEIGHBORHOOD HEALTH CENTER

Mission Neighborhood Health Center (MNHC) was opened in the late 1960s by the Office of Economic Opportunity, the War on Poverty's central agency, to provide health services to San Francisco's Mission District. More recently, MNHC has been funded by the federal Department of Health, Education and Welfare (HEW), which took over many of the War on Poverty programs. MNHC is the only fully bilingual health service available to the tens of thousands of non-English speaking Latino people of San Francisco.

During its first years, MNHC was run by a medical entrepreneur who used MNHC funds to help develop his own private medical office building nearby (Hartman and Feshback, 1974). In 1975, a months-long community struggle forced HEW to give the MNHC grant to the Mission Area Health Associates (MAHA), a new community group with a board of trustees whose majority was supposed to be elected by the health center's own patients. MAHA's victory was considered to be a triumph for community control at MNHC.

In 1977, a small clique of Latino youths gained control over the MAHA board of trustees. This clique ran a network of Mission District poverty agencies, mainly concerned with youth programs, including the Real Alternatives Program, Centro de Cambio and Mission Community Legal Defense. At MNHC they named another member of their clique to the $25,000 a year job as health center administrator, though their friend had no experience administering a health care institution.

By 1979 the health center was in shambles and its patients were up in arms. Patients were forced to wait in long lines to pay fees before being cared for. For several months, patients who had outstanding bills were not allowed to receive medical services until they settled their bills. Many patients were receiving incorrect bills for sevices they had never gotten or had already paid for. A number of competent health professionals and employees were terminated, sometimes leaving patients without their health care provider from one day to the next. The board had purchased an extremely expensive and poorly programmed computer that caused patients to wait an average of 1 3/4 hours to register at the health center. Transportation services for elderly patients were reduced while money was wasted on excess administrative salaries. The health center's financial deficit topped $200,000.[*]

Worst of all, the clique running the board refused to hold the yearly elections required by their own by-laws. As the San Francisco Examiner's columnist Guy Wright (1979a) put it,

> Board members whose terms expired more than a year ago still cling to their seats, adopting budgets, handing out raises, firing anyone who objects -- and appointing friends to fill vacancies when anyone resigns from the board.

HEW, which has the responsibility of administering the MNHC grant, knew of and ignored or encouraged the mismanagement at the health center. HEW allowed the health center's administrative costs to increase from 21 percent to 28 percent of the budget (U.S. Department of HEW, 1979a), though HEW suggests that such costs not exceed 20 percent. HEW approved the purchase of the computer that was later investigated by the FBI for possible fraudulent bidding practices and kickbacks (U.S. Department of HEW, 1979b). HEW allowed the clinic's board members to continue in office beyond their legal terms of office without demanding immediate elections, and HEW repeatedly backed this board as the health center's legitimate governing body.

THE HEALTH CENTER'S PATIENTS FIGHT BACK

In 1979, as a result of community pressure, new elections finally began. But in May, the clique controlling the board disqualified a number of the candidates in the election. Board members and their supporters physically and verbally intimidated volunteers attempting to help get the election underway. A fight took place at the clinic between board members and volunteers, and the election never took place.

Thereupon, seventy patients of the health center sued

---

[*]Documentation for the facts presented in this paragraph come from numerous MNHC memos and from the author's own experience of being employed at MNCH for 3½ years before his firing in June 1979.

the board and won a June 8 agreement that the elections
must start immediately, under the supervision of a
neutral third party. Still, no action was taken to hold
the elections. With the help of the Rebel Worker
Organization and the Grass Roots Alliance, worker and
community organizations who had been asked to get
involved, over 100 patients formed themselves into the
Patients Defense Association. They arrived en masse at
the June 20 MAHA board meeting to demand decisive
patient representation in the running of the clinic.
They were denied.

The Association, many of whose members were already
refusing to use clinic services, voted to formally
boycott the clinic. For four weeks, the patients
picketed the clinic, marching, educating and persuading.
Hundreds of patients honored the boycott, going without
health care or using alternative health services set up by
the Rebel Worker Organization. Patients sent hundreds of
letters and petition signatures to their elected representatives in Washington. By the end of the boycott, the
Patients Defense Association had grown to 800 members.

During the boycott, physical intimidation showed
itself again. One Patients Defense Association activist
had sugar poured into the gas tank of her car; another
had her car windshield broken; and yet another had
objects thrown at the windows of her home. Gangs of
youths threateningly drove around the picket line, which
was largely made up of women and children.

Finally, the Regional Health Administrator of HEW,
Dr. Sheridan Weinstein, met with the Patients Defense
Association and agreed to guarantee a fair election procedure. But at the same time that Dr. Weinstein was
negotiating with the Association, his office was
encouraging and financing a lawsuit against the very
organizations (the Grass Roots Alliance, Rebel Worker
Organization, and the Institute for the Study of Labor
and Economic Crisis) who were assisting the patients in
their struggle for democratic elections and decent health
care. This lawsuit, brought by the clique controlling
the MAHA board, asked for $1 million in damages for libel
and conspiracy.

HEW's promise to guarantee fair elections had little
substance. The Patients Defense Association's lawyers
were forced to go into court time and time again, and
only after obtaining ten court orders did the elections
finally take place. The MAHA board and its lawyers,
using HEW funds to finance one after another courtroom
maneuver, delayed the elections in every way possible,
including resisting a judge's order. HEW was clearly supporting the MAHA board and thereby keeping the organized
working class patients from participating in the election. Only another massive letter writing appeal to
government officials, combined with victory after victory

in court, brought about the elections. On October 9, after an intense five month struggle, the elections were concluded. All patients Defense Association candidates won seats on the new MAHA board by overwhelming majorities.

HEW again moved to block organized working class power over the clinic. After reducing the clinic's budget, HEW laid down strict conditions to the new board requiring immediate crippling layoffs of clinic employees and cutbacks in services. Failure to meet these conditions would result in the replacement of the new MAHA board by another community agency. The new board, with its patient majority, is faced with running a clinic left in financial shambles by the old board and beseiged by HEW cutbacks and threats to take the grant away. As columnist Guy Wright (1979b) put it,

> HEW, which gave the old board extra money because it was doing such a poor job, has cut back on funding for the new board, which must clean up the mess.

ANALYSIS: HEW AS COUNTERINSURGENCY

Historically, the federal government has spent money for welfare and social service programs only at times of mass insurgency by the working class (Piven and Cloward, 1971). In the 1930s the government enacted social security, unemployment and welfare programs in response to the demonstrations and protests of millions of people, many organized by the growing Communist Party. The 1950s, with little organized working class unrest, produced almost no new social programs. But the 1960s, with its civil rights movement and urban rebellions, brought a massive increase in welfare expenditures, new health programs including Medicare, Medicaid and neighborhood health centers, educational programs such as Headstart, and "community action" and legal services programs to put some pressure on local and state governents. In fact, many of the War on Poverty programs were targeted into areas of actual or potential urban rebellion.

These federal moneys, then, served as a massive domestic counterinsurgency effort, designed to stop any effective working class protest that could take root and threaten the stability of the existing capitalist order. Domestic counterinsurgency works by

1. channeling money to programs which minimally alleviate the worst horrors of life in minority working class communities but which principally provide charity and create dependency on government funds; and

64

> 2. funneling the money through agencies that hire
> working class leaders and buy them off with
> $20,000 a year positions and with control over
> other jobs in the community.

Those who would not be bought off in this manner were frequently assassinated or imprisoned, for example, leaders of the Black Panthers. Those who were coopted became known to many as poverty pimps, and formed a new stratum of society, a stratum created by the needs of the state to control the working class in minority neighborhoods (Rebel Worker Newsjournal, 1979). The poverty pimps became the managers of the counterinsurgency programs, and as such gained control over aspects of the lives of the working class majority in their communities. Their control was termed "community control: because the poverty pimps came from the community. In this sense, "community control" has come to mean control over the working class community. The clique that ran the MAHA board from 1977 to 1979 is a clear example of this stratum of poverty pimps.

THE POVERTY PIMPS: A LUMPEN PETTY BOURGEOISIE

Using the terminology of Marxist class analysis, the poverty pimps are a new stratum of the lower rungs of the bourgeois class. Our society is made up of two antagonistic classes, the bourgeoisie (capitalist class) and the proletariat (working class) (Dixon, 1979). The capitalist class owns and controls the vast majority of the wealth -- the land, the factories, the oil and natural resources. The working class is forced to work for the capitalist class in order to survive, and those unable to work become dependent upon and controlled by government programs such as social security, unemployment compensation, disability and such services as those offered by neighborhood health centers.

The lower strata of the bourgeois class are the petty (small) bourgeoisie, most of whom today are employed by capital or by the state as managers and professionals. Their function is to carry out the orders of the capitalists in controlling and commanding the day-to-day activities of the working class (Braverman, 1974). In the factory, this function is performed by the planners, managers and foremen; in the welfare system it is performed by the social workers. The petty bourgeoisie does not in itself possess control over the country's resources but, in return for financial rewards, it serves as a transmission belt of control between the bourgeoisie and the working class.

The stratum of the petty bourgeoisie that we call the poverty pimps is a new stratum, created by the counterinsurgency programs of the federal government. Their purpose is to manage these programs for the benefit of the government and there by to pacify and control the working class on behalf of the bourgeoisie. Many poverty pimps may have taken their poverty agency positions with the best of intentions. But any desires to serve the community are snuffed out by the reality that they function as part of a state apparatus designed to rule and control their communities (Rebel Worker Newsjournal, 1979). The poverty pimps have a stake in maintaining the status quo in order to keep their own jobs. They may engage in petty (or big) rip-offs of public funds, and they create well-paying jobs for their friends and themselves to preserve and expand their positions and control. They come to identify with the government funding agency against their own people.

When the poverty funds begin to shrink, the poverty pimps may resort to any means -- including using their own gangs -- to keep their jobs and their control and to prevent themselves from being forced back into the working class whence they came. This stratum of poverty pimps is actually a <u>lumpen</u> petty bourgeoisie*, a stratum of parasites created by the War on Poverty, supported by taxpayers' money.

To conceal their true purpose from the working class that they exploit, those poverty pimps who are from minority communities may use the ideology of nationalism; for example,

> How can you criticize me, I'm Raza. We are united by the racism we experience, so you should support me. It doesn't matter that I make $30,000 a year while you and your family are on welfare. We are the same because my name is Gomez too (Martinez, 1979).

This kind of nationalism is a trick against the working class. It takes people's hatred of racism and twists it into a weapon against them (Martinez, 1979). And many white liberal and progressive people glorify the poverty pimps, calling them "The Community," when actually they are a tiny portion of the community that exploits the working class majority.

Domestic counterinsurgency and its creation of a lumpen petty bourgeoisie is in essence no different than the international counterinsurgency which motivated such programs as the Alliance for Progress in the 1960s. The Alliance for progress infused money into Latin America to

---

*According to Marx, the <u>lumpen</u> proletariat are the petty criminals, pimps, small drug pushers -- the poor who steal from the poor and exploit the poor, whose role in history is as a "bribed tool of reactionary intrigue."

pacify growing anti-American social movements.* It also created and strengthened a stratum of compradors (people who sold out the interests of their country for personal gain) similar to the poverty pimps, to administer the Alliance for Progress money and to control the population (for descriptions of world class formation, see Dixon, 1978; Jonas and Dixon, 1979). In its arsenal of counterinsurgency techniques, the Alliance for Progress utilized both the carrot and the stick: the food, agricultural and housing programs; and the repressive military and police apparatus.

HEW domestic counterinsurgency also utilizes both the carrot and the stick. the carrot is the charity of giving money to tranquilize the people and buy off their leaders; to make people depend on welfare checks, food stamps and neighborhood health centers; and thereby to prevent their organizing to really change their situation in society. The trick is to take away these charities if people cause trouble, a stick which is used to control both the poverty pimps and the working class. "Step out of line and you'll lose your little empire," the Feds tell the pimps. "Step out of line and you'll lose your food stamps, your clinics or your Headstart programs," the pimps tell the people (Rebel Worker Newsjournal, 1979).

COUNTERINSURGENCY AT MISSION NEIGHBORHOOD HEALTH CENTER

At MNHC, HEW counterinsurgency has shown itself as unwavering support for the poverty pimps, the small clique that controlled the MAHA board, against the organized working class patients. HEW knew for months that the board was violating its own by-laws by not holding elections, yet HEW continued to back them. In particular, when the Patients Defense Association, Rebel Worker Organization and Grass Roots Alliance began to work together to demand fair elections, HEW financed and encouraged the board's legal maneuvers to sabotage the elections and to sue the patients' supporters (Puga v. Hernandez, 1979). HEW attempted to discourage the patients and make them give up, and on several occasions blamed the patients for causing the problems at the clinic, problems for which HEW was actually responsible. And in encouraging the lawsuit against the patients'

---

*The Alliance for Progress also served to create demand for U.S. products, which is an example of state capitalism -- taxpayers' money funneled into corporate profits. HEW funding of health programs is also state capitalist as well as counterinsurgent, but that is not the subject of this paper.

supporters, HEW was attempting to silence its own critics, showing no regard for freedom of speech and the
right of responsible criticism.

The clique running the MAHA board acted in classic
lumpen petty bourgeois fashion, with its financial
exploitation of the working class -- making the patients
pay increased clinic fees (often in cash) to support the
high administrative salaries voted by the board for their
friends. The clique did everything in its power to keep
the working class from taking away its control over the
clinic. And the clique attempted to disorganize the
patients by warning that further protest would cause HEW
to close down the clinic ("Step out of line and you'll
lose your clinic.")

Now that the clique has been removed and a new
patient-dominated board has been elected, HEW is pulling
out an old favorite in its bag of counterinsurgency tricks:
if you don't do what we say, we'll give the grant to
someone else ("Step out of line and you'll lose your
little empire.") In its October 3, 1979, grant award, HEW
places twenty conditions on the new board, in particular
the requirement for immediate substantial cutbacks in
services. If the new board fails to meet these anti-
patient conditions, HEW will look for another organization to run the clinic (U.S. Department of HEW, 1979c).
In that way, HEW is trying to repeat the cycle: trying to
turn a new group of working class people into a new clique
of poverty pimps, who take the side of HEW rather than of
the patients whom they were elected to represent. Using
the carrot (control over jobs and money) and the stick
(do what we want or we'll give the grant to someone
else), HEW will forever attempt to coopt and control the
struggles of working class people for a voice in the
decisions that affect their lives.

THE FIGHT FOR TRUE PATIENT REPRESENTATION

The struggle for elections at MNHC was not a
struggle to replace one set of poverty pimps with
another. It was about democracy, about a voice for the
majority of working class people in our country who have
always been disenfranchised and ignored. The patients who
won the recent MNHC election didn't seek to be on the
board as unaccountable individuals. They were chosen as
representatives of the 800-member Patients Defense
Association, and they pledged to represent the interests
of the Association, of the patients of the health center,
and not just of themselves.

In a statement made during the MNHC boycott, the
Patients Defense Association spoke:

For too long, patient representation has been a sham
at the health center. One set of so-called "community

leaders" after another have gained control, claiming the support of the community that they did not have. Until now, patients have never organized for the principle of true patient representation. If patients are not organized, these small groups of "leaders" can continue to get in power and refuse to listen to us. We are trying to do something that we haven't seen done before: get patient representatives who are accountable to a democratic organization of hundreds of patients (Patients Defense Assocation, 1979).

Whether true patient representation can actually be achieved in the case of MNHC remains to be seen. The counterinsurgent pressure from HEW is strong and must be resisted everyday. What counts is whether the new board will consistently fight for the interests of the patients and against the control imposed by HEW.

REFERENCES

Braverman, Harry
    1974   Labor and Monopoly Capital. New York: Monthly Review Press.
Davis, Karen and Cathy Schoen
    1978   Health and the War on Poverty: A Ten Year Appraisal. Washington: The Brookings Institution.
Dixon, Marlene
    1978   "Abstract: The Degradation of Waged Labor and Class Formation on an International Scale." Synthesis, Vol. II, No. 3 (Spring): 50.
    1979   In Defense of the Working Class. San Francisco: Synthesis Publications.
Hartman, C. and Dan Feshbach
    1974   "Mission District Health Hustle." Common Sense (December).
Jonas, Susanne and Marlene Dixon
    1979   "Proletarianization and Class Alliances in the Americas." Synthesis, Vol, III, No. 1 (Fall): 1.
Martinez, Betita
    1979   "White, Black or Brown: A Poverty Pimp is a Poverty Pimp." Rebel Worker Newsjournal (June).
Patients Defense Association
    1979   "The Fight for True Patient Representation."
Piven, Francis Fox and Richad A Cloward
    1971   Regulating the Poor: the Functions of Public Welfare. New York: Vintage Books.

Puga, V. Hernandez
    1979   Affidavits filed in the U.S. District Court, San Francisco, on September 7, 1979 by trustees, administrators and lawyers for MNHC.
Rebel Worker Newsjournal
    1979   "Who are our Friends and Who are our Enemies?" (June).
U.S. Department of Health Education and Welfare
    1979a   Program Indicators.
    1979b   Memo from Region IX HEW office to San Francisco office of the FBI.
    1979c   October 3 Notice of Grant Award to MNHC.
Wright, Guy
    1979a   "A Sick Health Center." San Francisco Examiner (August 1).
    1979b   "Health Center Future." San Francisco Examiner (November 22).

6
Veterans' Medical Care: The Politics of an American Government Health Service

Judith Lasker   Bucknell University

The history of veterans' benefits and services in the
United States is reviewed; it demonstrates their
responsiveness to dominant political, economic, military and medical interests. The ideological position
that social services must be "deserved" is also seen
to be an important influence on the V.A. system. The
consequent inaccessibility of V.A. medical care to
most veterans and almost all non-veterans raises
questions about the appropriateness of the V.A.
system as a model for national health care.

The vast and ever-increasing literature on medical
care in the United States all but ignores a major component of the national medical system--the medical services and institutions of the Veterans Administration.
Although the V.A. has the "largest medical-care delivery
system in the United States" (National Academy of Science,
1977: 1), it is rare to find it even mentioned in discussions of national health policies. However, when it is
mentioned in the literature, the V.A. is often discussed
as a model for a potential national health system (Lipsky
et al, 1976; Sapolsky, 1977; Chase, 1977). Since,
despite criticisms of its quality and relevance (National
Academy of Sciences, 1977; Starr, 1973), the V.A. is
likely to continue to be an important segment of American
health care in any type of future system, it is essential
to examine the model carefully. This paper reviews
available literature, the history of veterans' medical

I would like to thank Bucknell University for a grant
received to carry out this research. Thanks also to
Gregory Gaertner, Allen Imershein, Florence Datz, Arnold
Lasker, Miriam Lasker, John Kendrick, Jean Potuchek,
Matthew Silberman, Barry Siegel, Martha Verbrugge, Albert
Wesssen and the V.A. library staff for their helpful com-
ments and assistance.

services, and recently collected utilization data in order
to analyze the principles underlying the creation and
continued growth of the V.A. medical system. One must
examine the forces which have influenced this set of institutions if one wants to consider the possibilities for
a system of national health care in the United States.
     One can only conclude from the paucity of literature
that the V.A. medical system is considered an aberration
by most students of American health care (if it is considered at all)—a federally-run national health service
in a nation presumably dedicated to free enterprise medicine. This paper will present the proposition that the
V.A. medical system is not at all an abberation. Rather,
I suggest that it is very similar to other health and
social services in the United States. It consists of a
set of resources whose distribution and administration
have been subject to the priorities of dominant interests
in the society. Military, political, economic, and
medical elites have all participated in shaping medical
care for veterans. Although their efforts have produced
ever-improving and expanding services for millions of
people, their interests in the V.A. system go beyond the
goal of caring for veterans' medical problems. The other
priorities may in fact conflict with or detract from
the ideal of comprehensive, accessible, and high quality
health care. It is these other goals which will be considered in this paper.
     It will be necessary first to discuss this view of
social services as societal resources allocated to serve
goals other than those of meeting the needs of clients.
Secondly, the history of veterans' services will be examined as an example of this phenomenon, and the impact of
various interests on that history will be analyzed. An
additional factor which affects V.A. medicine and is
also significant in other social services is the ideological position that some potential clients are more
deserving of services than others. The specific characteristics of the hierarchy of eligibility are also
related to non-medical priorities. In the last section,
the effect these issues have on the ability of the V.A.
to meet the needs of its client population will be considered. The purpose here is to analyze the factors
which result in the inequitable distribution of national
social welfare resources. A national health system which
resembles the V.A. would potentially also be subject to
these same inequalities.

THE POLITICS OF SOCIAL SERVICES

     A number of authors over the last few years have exa-
mined health and social services in the U.S. and have
pointed out that they serve the economic and political
interests of dominant groups in the society. Foremost

among these analysts has been Vicente Navarro (1976, 1977a), who has demonstrated that ownership and/or control of medical services by the upper-class have produced a system which meets the needs of this small minority more than those of the majority of the populations. Krause examines the process by which health programs are subordinated to the goals of power and profit and how this is justified by the dominant capitalist ideology. He asserts that "...health care is simply one type of housekeeping function which a capitalist state needs to keep the wheels of industry rolling,...no understanding of the health service system is possible without looking outside of it to the wider political economy" (1977:154).

Studies of medical services in other societies have also revealed underlying interests which produce systems often unresponsive to the health problems of the population. For instance, Field's (1957) study of medical services in the Soviet Union during the Stalinist era of heavy industrialization showed the role of physicians in promoting economic growth by limiting the number of sick days available to workers. An analysis of health care in the Ivory Coast reveals the continuous use of medical resources, both during colonial rule and after independence, to promote economic growth and political stability (Lasker, 1977). An increasing number of studies on national health systems support this viewpoint (Navarro, 1977b).

When the state is directly involved in the planning and direction of health care services, as it is in most nations other than the United States, the impact of these other interests is most visible. Yet the same analysis can also be applied in the American context. Waitzkin and Navarro both note that the American government uses medical resources to reduce popular dissent, to provide profit for private industry, and to reinforce "dominant frameworks in scientific and clinical medicine that are consistent with the capitalist economic system" (Waitzkin, 1978: 36).

The state's support of economic and political goals through the distribution of medical resources is one aspect of its activities in the broader area of social welfare services. An number of scholars have pointed out the many ways in which American welfare policies respond to the dominant capitalist interests by promoting stability, maintaining a reserve of surplus labor, funding private enterprise (for instance, through housing programs) and reinforcing values of individualism (by stigmatizing recipients and eliminating from the rolls any who might be considered 'undeserving'). These priorities have shaped policy much more than any assessment of the needs of the nation's poor (Piven and Cloward, 1971; Galper, 1975).

The V.A. medical care system offers an important case

to illustrate the applicability of this analysis to medical care in the United States. It reflects both direct state involvement and the influence of the institutions and models of private medicine. It is funded and administered by the federal government but is closely tied to medical schools and the prevailing patterns of personnel training and hierarchy. Studying the history of the V.A. illuminates the significance of political, military, economic and organized medical interests in determining the characteristics of V.A. medical care.

V.A. MEDICAL CARE - HISTORICAL OVERVIEW[1]

Medical care was first made available to disabled veterans in the United States with the establishment of the Soldiers' Home, the Naval Home, and the National Homes for Disabled Volunteer Soldiers following the Civil War. Except for the men admitted to these few institutions, no other medical care was provided for veterans until World War I, when Public Health Service hospitals or private hospitals under contract with the Bureau of War Risk Insurance cared for the war-injured.

By 1920, fifty government hospitals were treating disabled soldiers and veterans, and Congress allocated funds for the construction of more hospitals. A Veterans' Bureau, created in 1921 to consolidate insurance and medical functions, took over the administration of the Public Health Service Hospitals which were serving veterans. In 1930, the Veterans Administration replaced the Veterans Bureau and incorporated the National Homes and the Bureau of Pensions. Since 1930, the V.A. system has continued to grow. It now operates 172 hospitals, 104 nursing homes and domiciliaries, and 220 outpatient clinics, employs 181,000 people, and has a budget for 1980 of $5.6 billion (Wehr, 1979a).

The growth of V.A. medical services has continued both in wartime and in peacetime, due to a different set of forces at work in each situation. During every war in this century, Congress has allocated increased funds for the care of the wounded. Each period of mobilization produced additional veterans and added to the numbers of the disabled. As a result, facilities were expanded and new ones built to accommodate the demand.

The number of disabled patients diminished, however, within a few years after each war, leaving the problem of unused hospital beds. The recent war having strengthened

---

[1]Unless otherwise indicated, historical information on veterans' medical care in this and other sections was drawn from two sources: Adkins, 1967, and Weber and Schmeckebier, 1934.

the V.A. structures and contributed to the ranks of veterans' organizations, political pressures were brought to bear on Congress to loosen eligibility requirements in order to increase admissions rather than cut back on facilities. By the time the next war started, the V.A. hospitals were again close to capacity, and Congress again allocated funds for additional facilities to accommodate the increased number of veterans and wounded soldiers. The result of this continual expansion in eligibility and beds is that, at present, only 17 percent of patients in V.A. hospitals are being treated for service-connected disabilities; most of the others are admitted on the basis of other criteria such as economic need (Cleland, 1979).

Despite the important influence of the V.A. and its employees, the veterans' organizations, and supporters in Congress, veterans' medical services have also come under attack from a wide variety of sources. Increase in access to these services for the non-disabled has been opposed by private medicine as unfairly competitive. The quality of care provided in veterans' institutions has been continuously challenged by journalists and scholars. Most recently there has been considerable debate within government over the possibility of merger between V.A. and private medical care. Proponents of this merger point to the fact that only in medical care does the V.A. provide direct services rather than helping the veterans to purchase from the private market place, as it does in education and housing. The possibility of national health insurance as well as criticisms of quality, cost, duplication of services, and difficulty of access have all fueled the controversy over the future of veterans' medical care. Nevertheless, the V.A. medical system has continued to grow and will certainly persist in the foreseeable future (cf. Lindsay, 1975).

INFLUENCES ON V.A. HEALTH CARE

Political Interests

The fact that political influence of different groups has played an important role in the development of the V.A. system is hardly surprising, since it is a creature of the legislative process. It is interesting, however, to examine the role of political influence in the expansion of facilities and benefits. The veterans' organizations (American Legion, Disabled American Veterans, Veterans of Foreign Wars, etc.) are the most intensely involved in influencing the political process, and veterans in Congress play a strategic role in the passage of legislation regarding the V.A.

The importance of political pressure from veterans is probably as old as the existence of benefits. In the fifteenth century, for example, when standing armies developed to serve feudal lords, disabled soldiers were cut off from community support, and they organized to demand redress. This pressure led to the formulation of a variety of pension plans and domiciliary homes. These plans were limited and mostly unsuccessful, but during the sixteenth and seventeenth centuries, the number of veterans' homes and assistance plans increased in Europe, and these were adopted in part by the American colonies.

Active organizing of veterans in the United States dates to the turn of this century. The United Spanish War Veterans was founded in 1898; Veterans of Foreign Wars was established in 1913. Both exerted pressure on Congress to expand benefits, and partly as a result of this pressure, both pension and medical benefits were greatly liberalized following World War I.

The effect of organized protest is also seen whenever efforts are made to cut back on benefits. In 1933 Congress passed a bill, proposed by President Roosevelt in response to Depression conditions, which drastically reduced pensions and services for vetreans. After massive protest and despite a presidential veto, Congress reversed itself in 1934. A similar result occurred in 1965 when a new V.A. administrator ordered the closing of some outmoded and underutilized hospitals and the building of new ones in other areas. Veterans' organizations, V.A. employees and Congressmen from the affected districts opposed the plan, resulting in a review and modification.

More recently, a report by the National Academy of Sciences on "Health Care for American Veterans," commissioned by Congress, created a great furor by proposing the gradual integration of V.A. medical facilities with the private medical sector, suggesting that a separate system is unnecessary. Members of Congress interested in veterans' affairs, many of whom are themselves veterans of military service, responded angrily by attacking the NAS study group and initiating an audit of its books by the General Accounting Office (Science, 1978).

According to an editorial in the New England Journal of Medicine (1978) commenting on the report's reception, "...the V.A. medical care system is a sacred cow. The whole subject is so loaded with political emotion and vested interests that rational public discourse is hardly possible." An editor of Science responded similarly: "The V.A., of course, has a unique clientele and a history of special treatment by Congress. There are roughly 28 million veterans who, with their families, constitute a potentially formidable voting bloc. Veterans' interests are championed by veterans' organizations which form a highly effective single interest lobby." In addition to these groups, the many families supported by jobs in the V.A. hospitals also have an interest in their continuation. The editorial concludes that the NAS study group had "triggered a powerful, protective, conditioned reflex" (<u>Science</u>, 1978).

The organized pressure of interested groups combined with the military service history of many powerful members of Congress has resulted in the continued expansion of services and benefits. For instance, recent legislation created counseling programs of Vietnam-era veterans, preventive health services for veterans with service-connected disabilities, and expanded medical services for dependents, and increased outpatient dental care. When two fiscally conservative senators challenged these expenditures in committee and succeeded in cutting the amount of money allocated in the bill by one-third, their action was quickly reversed by the Congress. The combined efforts of veterans' groups, the V.A. staff, and veterans in Congress has resulted in continual growth of such new programs and expansion of eligibility for existing programs (Wehr, 1979a, 1979b, 1979c; Crosby, 1979). Political influence has also played an important part in the location of facilities; a number of cities are the sites of V.A. hospitals because they were the home towns of an American president or of an influential member of Congress (Sapolsky, 1977: 373-4).

Despite evidence of their continued impact on legislation, leaders of veterans' organizations worry about what they consider to be a decline in their political influence. They point in particular to efforts by President Carter and the Office of Management and Budget to cut back on medical personnel, facilities and benefits in order to save money. The decreasing proportion of members of Congress with military service histories and the fading of public support for veterans, especially after Vietnam, have made the V.A. increasingly vulnerable to the actions of budget-conscious officials (Estill, 1979; Wehr, 1979d). According to the Twentieth Century Fund Task Force on Policies toward Veterans, the strength of the veterans' organizations has decreased steadily since the 1950s because of the lack of participation of younger veterans. Nevertheless, "Theirs is virtually the only point of view ever expressed before the congressional veterans committees...no countervailing political force has yet managed to dispute effectively the view of the veterans' organizations." The report concludes that future Congressional response to organized veterans' demands is "hard to predict" (Taussig, 1974: 57-9). The dependence of medical services on political interests has up until now usually worked to the advantage of the V.A. system as a whole, but it may also ultimately lead to the curtailment of those services.

Military Interests

Educational, financial, and employment benefits have all been used in the U.S., as elsewhere, to induce military enlistments. Historically, one major incentive for men to become soldiers has been the reward of plunder and some times even parts of the conquered territories. Other kinds of state-sponsored rewards also served as incentives to fight. The ancient Greeks freed helots who offered distinguished service and also fed and pensioned disabled soldiers. An English law passed in 1592 to provide "for the Reliefe of Souldiours" offered pensions to the disabled "to the end that they may reap the fruit of their good deservings, and that others may be encouraged to perform the like endeavors." This latter intent was reflected in legislation passed in the American colonies. New Hampshire in 1718 legislated medical care for disabled veterans "for the better encouragement of soldiers to adventure their persons against the enemy." George Washington, after initially opposing service pensions for officers during the Revolutionary War, later changed his mind when many officers deserted the ranks, and he wrote to the Continental Congress asking for pensions in order to be able to keep enough officers to win the war.

When the first peacetime conscription was established by Congress in 1940, the bill included a variety of benefits for veterans, intended in part to reduce opposition to the draft. Men were reluctant to give up their jobs during a time of high unemployment, and the promise of government assistance after their release from service was offered as an incentive to assure the success of conscription. The G.I. Bill of 1944 was built upon these earlier provisions (Olson, 1974).

Economic Interests

Some of the efforts made to encourage enlistment have also been designed to assist the economy. For instance, in the nineteenth century, frontier lands were awarded to veterans, in part as a way to promote the frontier regions of the country. During the Depression, $3.5 million in adjusted benefits were awarded to World War I veterans, and this was seen as a way of stimulating the weakened economy. The G.I. Bill of 1944 was viewed not only as a reward to soldiers for military service but also as a mechanism for supporting the American educational system and the economy. According to Olson (1974), educational and financial benefits were enacted due to the fear that the reentry of veterans in great numbers into a shaky economy after the war would create massive unemployment and consequently dangerous political instability. The resulting advantage to individual veterans may be seen in the fact that their median income in 1977 was $4500 higher than that of non-veterans. The average educational attainment of veterans is higher than that of non-veterans, and at each educational level veterans have higher incomes (Cleland, 1979). Preference given to veterans in civil service hiring has certainly contributed to this advantageous position.

The building of V.A. medical facilities constitutes an important investment in a community and therefore may also be used as an economic tool. A recent decision to build a new V.A. hosptal in Camden, N.J. despite the existence of facilities in nearby Philadelphia, resulted from persistent political pressure on President Carter, who reversed his opposition to the plan. Camden's mayor described the project as "the cornerstone of a rebuilding program intended to restore the city's economic viability." The hospital was expected to generate 1000 jobs directly and many more indirectly because of the growth of doctors' offices, restaurants, bank branches, and other business (New York Times, Feb. 22, 1978).

The V.A. system has also contributed to the economic well-being of professional interests. Medical schools, for instance, have found V.A. hospitals to be a useful source of "teaching material," research funds, and additional teaching staff (Sapolsky, 1977). In 1978, the V.A. had 2000 arrangements with schools teaching health professionals, and more than 97,000 students received training in V.A. facilities (Cleland, 1979). The Camden V.A. Hospital, for instance, was planned in conjunction with the expansion of a private medical center to include training of medical students.

Organized Medical Interests

Despite these economic and teaching advantages, one would expect organized medical interests to oppose the expansion of V.A. services. The AMA, for instance, has waged a battle against state-funded or administered medical care for decades (Burrow, 1963; Marmor, 1970; Stevens, 1971). Yet the V.A. has received considerable assistance and support from the AMA and from prominent medical educators. Since 1924, advisory groups of physicians from a broad range of specialty areas have been formed to assist the veterans' medical system. The first of these, the Medical Council, was chaired by Dr. Ray Lyman Wilbur, at that time President of Stanford University and also President of the AMA. The Secretary was Dr. Malcolm MacEachern, Associate Director of the American College of Surgeons, and the other officers were medical school professors. The Council endorsed the establishment of relations between V.A. hospitals and medical schools and the carrying out of medical research by the V.A.

Formal affiliation with medical schools was authorized

in 1946, and it has been seen as a major factor in up-grading the quality of V.A. medical care (National Academy of Sciences, 1977: 253). This relationship has been applauded both by the American Association of Medical Colleges and the editors of the Journal of Medical Education (JME, 1977). Adkins concluded that the "V.A. has the cooperation of organized medicine and an excellent reputation" (1967: 220).

The alliance with medical schools, however, has also been strongly criticized. It has resulted, according to some scholars, in the abandonment of the needs of the V.A.'s primary clientele--the chronically disabled, both physically and mentally--for the attractions of acute tertiary care and teaching (Lipsky, et al, 1976; Sapolsky, 1977).

Despite this history of cooperation, organized medical interests did oppose some facets of V.A. expansion, in particular, the inclusion of non-service connected veterans. The provision of general medical care for these patients more clearly intruded into the domain of private medicine. During the post-World War II period of V.A. reorganization, the AMA House of Delegates passed a resolution expressing its "long-estabished opposition to any attempt at the socialization of medicine in America by extending medical benefits under the Veterans Administration to encompass disabilities that are not service-connected or to general medical care of the dependents of veterans" (Starr, 1973: 75). Starr concludes that this ongoing opposition significantly slowed the development of V.A. health services and that the more recent extension of benefits (outpatient care for non-service connected veterans and services for some dependents) may be attributed to a decline in AMA power.

Ideological Component

The history of social welfare is permeated by repeated attempts to separate the "deserving" from the "undeserving" and to provide benefits only for the former. Legislators as well as private agencies have sought to make assistance available only to those whom they have determined not to be personally at fault for their misfortune, particularly children, the elderly, the disabled, and widows. Able-bodied men have rarely received aid because, except in cases of severe national depression or disruption, they have been assumed to be responsible for their own suffering. This idea of indi-vidual responsibility is a strong ideological component of capitalism and a persistent theme in public opinion and in social policy (Rimlinger, 1971; Feagin, 1975; Galper, 1975). Its consequence is the limitation of assistance only to those who demonstrate exceptional cir-cumstances or merit.

The veteran, and especially the disabled veteran, is an excellent example of this principle. He (and in 98 percent of cases the veteran is a male) has been treated not only as the victim of exceptional circumstances but is doubly deserving for having served the country in battle. He has therefore "earned" the right to a variety of benefits, including education, employment advantages, and medical care.

Robinson Adkins, a V.A. official and the author of a history of veterans' medical care, wrote, "The American people, acting through Congress, have supported the principle that a man who devotes part of his life--usually his young manhood--to defend his country, should be offered advantages over those who do not" (1967: 4). The principle of rewarding those who have served in the military is a very old one. In ancient Rome, municipal offices were often awarded to veterans and their descendants. Throughout the Middle Ages, various forms of cash relief and institutional care were provided for veterans. During the nineteenth century in the United States, veterans received free land as well as pension benefits. In 1917, when Secretary of the Treasury McAdoo transmitted to President Wilson legislation expanding veterans' benefits, he wrote, "Every man should know that the moment he is enlisted in the military service of the Government these definite guarantees and assurances are given to him, not as charity but as part of his deserved compensation for the extra hazardous occupation into which the Government has forced him" (Adkins, 1967: 94). Most recently, in response to proposals that the V.A. medical system be phased out, an economist commented that this would deprive many needy veterans--the elderly, poor, and chronically ill--of access to medical care (Ginzberg, 1978). The underlying assumption appears to be that these categories of people are more entitled to such care if they are veterans.

The provision of services to veterans is thus based on the notion that they have deserved it. The distinction according to merit is also found even within the veteran population. The most basic differentiation among veterans is between those with service-connected disabilities and those who were not disabled as a result of military service. This distinction has governed pension and compensation benefits since these were first voted in the U.S. in 1776 for disabled Revolutionary War soldiers. Although eligibility for medical care has been constantly redefined to include more veterans and more kinds of services, service-connected disability has remained the principle guarantee of care. Since 1924 financial need has also been considered a basis for hospital care if beds are available. Outpatient care, available originally only for service-connected disabilities, was extended in 1973 to veterans without disabilities if they are eligible for hospitalization and if such care is related to or would prevent hospitalization. Disabled veterans are subject to the same limitations if they seek outpatient treatment for a condition not related to their disability. Veterans without service-connected disabilities may also be hospitalized if they are 65 or older or if they are Medal of Honor winners. An honorable discharge and at least one day of active duty are prerequisites for any health care (National Academy of Sciences, 1977).

The eligibility criteria which must be met by applicants for V.A. medical care are increasingly complex. Each time that Congress enacts new medical benefits, it sets restrictions on categories of veterans who are eligible for them, and a priority ranking establishing who should be admitted first in case of insufficient facilities. For instance, dental benefits were extended in 1979 to veterans of the two World Wars and Korea, the totally disabled, and Vietnam veterans who had been prisoners of war for more than six months. At the same time, World War I veterans were accorded top priority ranking for access to outpatient medical services (Wehr, 1979c, 1979d).

Each year, approximately 20 percent of all applications for medical services are rejected as ineligible or not in need of care (Cleland, 1977, 1978, 1979). Only 10-13 percent of veterans use V.A. health services, suggesting that the large majority never apply. The priority system was created by Congress specifically to limit access to V.A. health care, and it certainly is one important factor in reducing utilization. Many veterans do not use V.A. facilities either because they are ineligible or because they mistakenly think they are. In a recent survey of rural veterans, the failure to use V.A. medical care was often explained as resulting from uncertainty about eligibility. The essential point is that eligibility, not need, governs access to V.A. system. This principle is characteristic of other health and welfare services.

IMPACT ON DISTRIBUTION

The limitation of governmentally-run services to "deserving" groups, the importance of political and economic forces in determining where facilities will be built, and the use of health services to promote military aims, all have the effect of exacerbating inequities in the U.S. medical care system. In particular, rural residents and women are at a disadvantage, the former because of inaccessibility of services, the latter because of eligibility requirements. Whenever medical resources are allocated by the state for purposes other than the alleviation of suffering and on bases other than need, the result is inequality in the availability of services to potential patients.

The distribution of 172 hospitals in a country the size of the United States inevitably leads to difficulties of access for many eligible veterans. Since distance is generally related to the use of medical services (Shannon et al, 1969), it is not surprising that rural veterans are much less likely to take advantage of their medical eligibility. A study of the use of services by veterans living on Cape Cod, for example, showed that the hour and half to three hours traveling time to a V.A. hospital inhibited its utilization. A review of outpatient records at the Providence V.A. Hospital, which serves Cape Cod as part of its region, revealed that only 1.1 percent of visits between March 1 and June 30, 1976 were by veterans from the Cape. Yet the veteran population on Cape Cod constitutes 8 percent of the veterans in the Providence region. A survey of veterans on Cape Cod revealed an almost total lack of use of V.A. medical facilities (Wessen et al, 1976). In a recent survey of 200 men in three rural counties in Central Pennsylvania, a similar failure to use any V.A. services was found.

Medical services for veterans, as with social and health services generally, begin and expand or contract in reponse to the organized political activity of client groups, legislators, the military, and those provider groups who might either benefit or suffer from greater involvement of the state. Consequently, services are often maldistributed or inappropriate. The location of hospitals has been decided on the basis of prestige needs of powerful leaders or lobbying abilities of local communities and their representatives rather than on an assessment of need. (The V.A. has so far been exempt from the certificate of need regulations governing private medical facilities).

CONCLUSION

Navarro writes that the American health care system reflects the class structure of U.S. society in its organization and in the decision-making process. Veterans' benefits, medical care being a major portion, may be analyzed similarly. They are neither an anomaly nor an anachronism. They directly respond to the economic, military and political priorities of powerful groups in the society. The fact that V.A. health services are federally financed and organized, not unlike the health systems of Eastern Europe, hardly means that socialism is rampant in the American government. It suggests rather that military goals are central to the society and, that, as a result, veterans are a powerful lobby and have the support of much of the population in their efforts to expand "well-earned" benefits. The V.A. system dramatically supports the dominant American value that services are a privilege to be earned and not a right of citizenship. This is certainly not a socialist approach. In addition, the care of aging, poor, and chronically disabled soldiers is generally uninteresting and unprofitable for the acute-care oriented practitioners who dominate private medicine, and they have not sought to take on this responsibility.

A national health system modeled on the V.A. may reflect the same principles and produce the same results. This would particularly be the case if national health care coexists with the private system, the former covering only special categories of people and those who are uninteresting to or cannot afford private medical care. Competition between the two systems for money and personnel has created some disadvantages for the V.A., since the resources of private medicine are so much greater (Starr, 1973). Continued coexistence of the two systems will perpetuate the weaknesses of the public services, as has already been seen in cities where public and private hospitals exist side by side (Kotelchuck, 1976).

The V.A. medical system has often benefited from the interests discussed here, but it is also vulnerable because of them. Unfavorable public reactions to the Vietnam War have diminished the "deserving" aura around its veterans, and thus weakened popular commitment to veterans' services. The reduction in numbers of veterans in Congress and the "deep generational divisions" between veterans of Vietnam and of earlier wars over the form that benefits should take (Wehr, 1979a) have resulted in attenuated political influence. In addition, budgetary concerns have led members of Congress to challenge the expenditure of funds for veterans as being too costly (Wehr, 1979b).

Certainly the V.A. medical system has provided much-needed care for millions of people. However, a study of the V.A. provides further evidence that societal resources are not distributed in response to universalistic principles of medical necessity (nor of economic efficiency). The predominance of other goals may present problems for many veterans (e.g. those in rural areas) as well as for non-veterans, who are excluded from this potentially important source of medical care.

REFERENCES

Adkins, Robinson
    1967   Medical Care of Veterans. Committee on Veterans' Affairs: U.S. Congress.
Burrow, James
    1963   AMA: Voice of American Medicine. Baltimore: Johns Hopkins Press.

Chase, John
     1977   "The V.A. Health Care Delivery System and
               National Health Insurance," Alabama Journal
               of Medical Science 14: 369-373.
Cleland, Max
     1977   Annual   Report   1976.   Washington,   D.C.:
               Administrator of Veterans Affairs.
     1978   Annual   Report   1977.   Washington,   D.C.:
               Administrator of Veterans Affairs.
     1979   Annual   Report   1978.   Washington,   D.C.:
               Administrator of Veterans Affairs.
Crosby, Imani
     1979   "Spending Increased for Veterans' Benefits."
               Congressional Quarterly Weekly Bulletin (Jan
               7): 134.
Estill, Robert
     1979   "Veterans Lose Clout in D.C.."   Bloomsburg,
               PA: The Morning Press (November 22): 15.
Feagin, Joe
     1975   Subordinating the Poor; Welfare and American
               Beliefs.   Englewood Cliffs, New Jersey:
               Prentice-Hall.
Field, Mark
     1957   Doctor   and   Patient   in   Soviet   Russia.
               Cambridge: Harvard University Press.
Galper, Jeffrey
     1975   Politics   of   Social   Services.   Englewood
               Cliffs, New Jersey: Prentice-Hall.
Ginzberg, Eli
     1978   "The NAS Report on the V.A.: How Not to
               Offer Congress Advice on Health Policy."
               New England Journal of Medicine 298 (March
               16): 11.
Journal of Medical Education
     1977   "The V.A.-Medical School Relationship." 52:1.
Kotelchuck, David
     1976   Prognosis Negative; Crisis in the Health Care
               System. New York: Vintage.
Krause, Elliot
     1977   Power and Illness: The Political Sociology
               of Health and Medical Care.   New York:
               Elsevier.
Lasker, Judith
     1977   "The Role of Health Services in Colonial
               Rule." Culture, Medicine, and Psychiatry 1:
               277-297.
Lindsay, Cotton
     1975   Veterans   Administration   Hospitals;   An
               Economic Analysis of Government Enterprise.
               Washington,   D.C.:   American   Enterprise
               Institute for Economic Research.

86

Lipsky, Michael, Lawrence McCray, Jeffrey Prottas, and Harvey Sapolsky
    1976   "The Future of the Veterans' Health Care System." Journal of Health, Politics, Policy, and Law 1 (Fall): 285-294.

Marmor, Theodore
    1970   The Politics of Medicare. Chicago: Aldine.

National Academy of Sciences
    1977   Study of Health Care of American Veterans. Washington, D.C.

Navarro, Vicente
    1976   Medicine under Capitalism. New York: Prodist
    1977a   "Social Class, Political Power and the State and their Implications in Medicine," International Journal of Health Services 7: 255-292.
    1977b   Social Security and Medicine in the USSR. Lexington, Mass: Lexington Books.

New England Journal of Medicine
    1978   "The Future of the Veterans Administration Hospital System: Two Points of View," 298 (March 16): 11.

New York Times
    1978   February 22: 51. (New Jersey).

Olson, Keith
    1974   The G.I. Bill, the Veterans, and the Colleges. Lexington: University Press of Kentucky.

Piven, Frances Fox, and Richard Cloward
    1971   Regulating the Poor: The Functions of Public Welfare. New York: Pantheon.

Rimlinger, Gaston
    1971   Welfare Policy and Industrialization in Europe, America, and Russia. New York: John Wiley.

Sapolsky, Harvey
    1977   "America's Socialized Medicine: The Allocation of Resources Within the Veterans' Health Care System." Public Policy 24 (Summer): 3.

Science
    1978   Editorial, Vol. 199 (March 3): 952-956.

Shannon, Gary et al.
    1969   "The Concept of Distance as a Factor in Accessibility and Utilization of Health Care." Medical Care Review 26 (February): 143-161.

Starr, Paul
    1973   The Discarded Army; Veterans after Vietnam. New York: Charterhouse.

Stevens, Rosemary
    1971   American Medicine and the Public Interest. New Haven: Yale U. Press.

Taussig, Michael
    1974   Those Who Served. Twentieth Century Fund Task Force on Policies toward Veterans. New York: Twentieth Century Fund.

Waitzkin, Howard
    1978   "A Marxist View of Medical Care." Science for the People 10 (Nov/Dec): 31-24.

Weber, Gustavius A. and Laurence Schmeckeier
    1934   The Veterans Administration; Its History, Activities and Organization. Service Monographs of the U.S. Government No. 66. Washington, D.C.: Brookings.

Wehr, Elizabeth
    1979a   "Freshman Senators Stall Veterans' Health Bill." Congressional Quarterly Weekly Bulletin. February 17: 297-8.
    1979b   "Spending Levels Chopped in Veterans' Health Bill." Congressional Quarterly Weekly Bulletin. March 17: 477-8.
    1979c   "Psychological Aid for Vietnam Vets Approved." Congressional Quarterly Weekly Bulletin. May 26: 1015-1017.
    1979d   "Carter Efforts to Cut V.A. Hospital Staffs Opposed." Congressional Quarterly Weekly Bulletin. June 23: 1251-2.

Wessen, Albert, Judith Lasker and Richard Fortinsky
    1976   "Report to Veterans Administration on Health Needs and Activities of Cape Cod Veterans." Mimeo.

7
Changing Physician Ideologies on the Care of the Dying: Themes and Possible Explanations

John MacDougall   University of Lowell

An analysis of changing physician ideologies regarding the care of elderly dying patients, as expressed in technical journals read by American physicians. Markedly more titles concerning terminal care are found in Index Medicus in 1968-78 than in 1960-67. In one journal, physicians are only after 1964 urged to tell patients openly about their condition and after 1969, to improve cooperation within professional teams. Two explanations of these data are tentatively explored: 1) a Parsonian explanation, whereby medical ideologies reflect professional autonomy and the influence of internalized moral norms; 2) a Marxist explanation, whereby medical ideologies reflect physicians' transformation from independent entrepreneurs into technological/bureaucratic agents of the state under monopoly captialism. Data are summarized which fail to support the Parsonian explanation, but which do support the Marxist explanation concerning the growth in salary payment of doctors and the government's role in terminal care.

INTRODUCTION

This chapter has two goals; first, to describe how the American medical profession has in recent years publicly stated its norms about the care of the elderly dying; and second, to explore in a preliminary way possible reasons for changes in these norms.[1]

Many thanks are due to Phil Brown, Johannes Fabian, Renee Fox, Liz Markson, Al Plough, Susan Reverby, and Irving Zola for their helpful comments, and to Sandra Abbott, Jill Clayton, Collette Destours, Carol Montgomery and Kathy Mull for research and clerical assistance.
[1]We only focus on the care of the aged dying. In the case of children, youths or relatively youthful adults who are dying, a different set of values are involved. (Parsons and Lidz, 1967).

The analysis in this paper is necessarily tentative and preliminay. There is to this author's knowledge no systematic analysis of changes in institutionalized medical ideologies regarding terminal care. Furthermore, there are few careful accounts of changing medical ideologies on any topic. Yet the topic of physician ideologies is important in understanding health-care in contemporary America. For physicians play a vital role not only in shaping everyday actions and expectations, but also in influencing national and regional resource allocations and decision-making procedures in health care. (MacDougall and Rawnsley, 1978).

An ideology may be defined as a set of interrelated cognitive perceptions and moral prescriptions/prohibitions pertaining to some social group. (Wallace, 1956; Waterman and Waitzkin, unpublished). In this chapter, our main concern is with the moral aspect of physicians' ideologies. The medical profession sees its work as based on modern science, yet always directed to the solution of practical problems.[2]

In the next section of this chapter, we describe some of the changes in physicians' ideologies since the 1950s, especially the greater salience of the whole issue of terminal care after 1967 and the increased emphasis in the later period on professional teamwork and on open discussions with patients. In Section III we briefly present three important perspectives in medical sociology. We then biefly review some data that will help us choose between those perspectives in explaining changes in medical ideologies after 1967. In Sections III and IV we suggest some ways in which a more rigorous analysis might be conducted.

THE NATURE OF IDEOLOGICAL CHANGES

An appropriate place to seek evidence of official medical ideologies is in professional medical journals. This is because the medical profession claims to be guided by general norms, scientific knowledge and practical expertise, and information on those matters is supposed to be public. Moreover, knowledge, experience and environmental conditions are always changing, and the medical profession is supposed to be adaptable and up-to-date, so doctors are expected to keep themselves informed

---

[2]Something may be learned about medical ideologies from the numerous studies of physicians' attitudes to death and dying. (e.g., Crane, 1975; Okin, 1961; Schulz and Aderman, 1976). However, such attitudes are not the same as ideologies, as we have defined the term, and most attitude studies fail to deal with the societal setting or with possible secular changes in attitudes.

about the latest scientific, practical and ethical developments.

Let us now consider evidence to be found in specific medical journals.

Numbers of Journal Articles

First, let us consider the frequency of entries on terminal care in Cumulated Index Medicus each year between 1960 and 1978. We have counted numbers of articles, editorials and letters on non-technical aspects of physicians' roles in the care of the aged dying.[3] These figures (Table 7.1) show that while the number of entries fluctuated quite sharply from year to year, the number was consistently higher after 1966 than before it.[4]

TABLE 7.1
Annual Numbers of Entries on the Care of the Dying Listed in Cumulated Index Medicus, 1960-77

Year	Number of Entries	Year	Number of Entries
1960	6	1970	18
1961	4	1971	26
1962	4	1972	20
1963	5	1973	29
1964	9	1974	22
1965	10	1975	14
1966	7	1976	29
1967	16	1977	18
1968	32*	1978	33
1969	12		

*Includes ten entries in Medical Times, which is an exceptionally large number of entries in one medical journal in one year.

Themes in Particular Medical Journals

To provide a qualitative description of changing medical ideologies, material in one particular medical journal has been subjected to content analysis. This

[3]Further details on methods of data-collection and analysis are available from the author.
[4]Year-to-year changes in numbers of articles in Index Medicus partly relect specific short-run developments like well-known lawsuits or new techniques. These changes are not considered in this paper.

journal is the Journal of Chronic Diseases (JCD for
short), a journal of considerable stature in the profession, whose contributors and editors represent specialties closely involved in the care of dying patients.
The JCD, since its establishment in 1955, has demonstrated a keen awareness of ethical and policy issues in
patient care, and a willingness to editorialize on those
issues. Thus statements in the JCD may be taken as quite
representative of the views of influential physicians and
of major centers of medical teaching and research on a
wide range of terminal-care issues.[5]

Table 7.2 shows that in no year was there a great
number of statements. However, there were markedly more
statements in 1969 and following four years, than before
1969.

TABLE 7.2
Annual Numbers of Statements on the Care of the Dying in
the Journal of Chronic Diseases, 1955-77

Year	Number of Statements	Year	Number of Statements
1955	1	1967	0
1956	0	1968	0
1957	0	1969	7
1958	3	1970	6
1959	0	1971	5
1960	0	1972	0
1961	0	1973	10
1962	0	1974	0
1963	10*	1975	0
1964	6	1976	0
1965	0	1977	1
1966	0		

*These statements were found in three articles or edi-
torials. In all other years in which statements on the
care of the dying were found, they were found in only one
article or editorial.

The themes of these statements were to some extent
different in the two sub-periods 1955-64 and 1969-77.
But there were also continuities between the two sub-
periods. Let us consider the most common themes.

[5]Statements in the JCD were drawn from all articles, editorials and letters that had to do with the care of dying
patients, or the care of sufferers from any chronic
disease.

The patient and his/her family. Both before and after 1969 it was often emphasized that doctors should control the patient's pain and distress. For example, it was suggested in 1973 that:

> the...objectives [of care for cancer patients in whom there is still obvious residual tumor growth left, even following primary treatment] may be defined as attempting to alleviate his symptoms so that the remaining period of the patient's life will be as comfortable and functional as possible, so that in the final period of his life no man should feel in today's society that he has been cast out to die. (Iszak et al, 1973: 371; cf. Hinton, 1964).

Another common point in the JCD is that physicians should pay closer attention to patients' emotional problems. In 1963, Dr. R. A. Senescu stated:

> Of particular importance in patients with acute emotional disturbance who may not have much time to live is the fact that...the problem was [and clearly, in Dr. Senescu's opinion, should be] dealt with directly and entirely in terms of the patient's present emotional reaction (Senescu, 1963: 830; cf. Theologides, 1971).

Concerning the intractable problems of what the physician should tell the dying patient and how, writers in the JCD continually emphasized the need for sympathy in discussions with the patient.[6] However, there are marked changes over time in opinions as to how openly the doctor should tell the patient he/she is dying. On this matter, a change of opinion occurred before the usual transitional year 1969. In 1958, Dr. R.R. Newell recommended:

> Don't try to tell [the patient] what you know he cannot accept...Don't tell him your diagnosis until you are sure...Manage to see mother (or wife, or husband) alone and quietly for an hour without the patient's knowing of it. Lie to the patient, if you must, for his own good...Leave the patient always one straw of hope to cling to. (Newell, 1958: 56-57).

---

[6]Okun (1961), commenting on his well-known study in the Journal of the AMA, felt that doctors should not tell patients about their condition. In the New England Journal of Medicine of 1957, the degradation of the patient by the modern slow method of dying is deplored. Yet it is never suggested that the problem might be alleviated by the frank discussion between doctor and patient (Life-in-Death, 1957).

Earlier in the article Dr. Newell said:

> At the very least you can ask the patient to look at
> the rapid advances of medical science and to hope
> that the cure for his disease is on the verge of
> discovery and will possibly be announced next week
> (Newell, 1958: 56).

But in an editorial in 1964, Dr. John Hinton urged
physicians to "speak more openly to dying patients and
their families" and to have a "quiet unhurried discussion
with the patient" (Hinton, 1964: 203). In 1969 Dr. Louis
Lasagna went further. Like Dr. Newell in 1958, Dr.
Lasagna advocated leaving some hope in the patient's
mind. But in all other respects, Dr. Lasagna disagreed
with Dr. Newell:

> While the patient has a right to live, he also has
> the right to die... In any case, the "truth" should
> always be told in a sympathetic and considerate
> manner, holding out at least some hope of the
> doctor's ability to modify certain manifestations of
> the disease, and to ease the pain or other distress.

> Lying to a patient about a serious illness is usually
> bad business, if for no other reason than that the
> patient will inevitably receive cues and clues about
> the truth from the environment (Lasagna, 1969: 67).

Relationships with colleagues. In the entire period
under discussion, articles and editorials in the JCD
advocated a team approach to terminal care. However,
different specific aspects of teamwork were mentioned in
1955-64 and in 1969-73. In the former period, teams were
discussed only in general terms (e.g., Conner et al,
1955). But in the 1970s, the contributions of specific
types of colleagues are mentioned--in positive tones.
These include priests and primary-care physicians (Iszak
et al, 1973; Theologides, 1971).

Moreover, the main problem in relationships with
colleagues that is mentioned in the 1950s and early 1960s
is group morale (Conner et al, 1955). But in the late
1960s and 1970s, cooperation and communications with
other physicians, nurses and social workers were seen as
seriously deficient (Iszak et al, 1973).

Thus in the late 1960s there emerged an emphasis on
greater honesty in relationships with patients, and on
closer collaboration with specific groups of professionals in the care of the dying.

EXPLANATIONS OF CHANGING IDEOLOGIES--A PRELIMINARY ANALYSIS

Parsons, Marx, and Freidson: General Models

Before attempting to explain the data just presented, let us summarize three sociological perspectives on the medical profession that are influential yet often incompatible.

The first is the Parsonian perspective, according to which doctors are influenced above all by their high moral and scientific standards, and have much autonomous control over the normative, scientific and technological aspects of their work. Physicians, it is argued, play an increasingly important role in propagating and implementing the instrumental-activist values of American society, especially as they relate to human life. Certain aspects and stages of life--of which death and dying are notable examples--cause much pain and uncertainty, owing to the advances of biomedical technology and to the secularization of American culture. Doctors are then called upon to make authoritative factual and normative statements, which are the functional equivalent of religious creeds and rules.[7]

Regarding the care of the dying, Parsons and his associates claim that physicians are influenced by both the public's demand for certainty and their own guilt at the prospect of "failure" when a patient dies. Because of these pressures, physicians seek first, to reinterpret the ancient Judeo-Christian value of the dignity and importance of divinely-given human life, in a new, relativistic form; and second, to formulate technical and ethical principles that justify the treatment of each individual patient. (Parsons, 1972; Parsons and Lidz, 1976: Parsons et al., 1973; Merton et al., 1957).[8]

The second perspective examined is the Marxist one, which sees the medical profession as gradually turning into agents of monopoly capital and its state apparatus. This is a complex dialectical process, but its main elements are the following.

The health-care industry is seen by Marxists as having

---

[7]Cf. Parsons' suggestion that health-care institutions are increasingly interested in mental illness, as somatic diseases come to be "conquered", and as greater responsibility is placed on the individual in a highly urbanized society (Parsons, 1972: 121). Parsons presumably feels that psychological problems pose very important challenges in terminal care.

[8]In particular, Parsons and Lidz (1967: 138) claim that physicians are expected to do everything possible to prevent deaths from being "premature" or "avoidable."

in the past two decades undergone a major change in its
mode of production, from a petty-commodity mode to a
large-scale, high-technology mode. Further, various
significant social and political changes have taken place
in recent years, largely to facilitate the change in the
mode of production. Most important, medicine has developed tighter links with profit making manufacturers of
drugs, supplies and equipment, more rigorous controls
over subordinate health care workers, and closer ties
with third-party payers (so as to ensure physicians'
solvency and continuous expansion of health-care institutions such as hospitals). Doctors and the organizations
where they work have also recently taken a closer
interest in state policy, and obtained larger amounts of
state funds. Doctors have done this both to promote the
above-mentioned relationships with manufacturers, subordinate workers, etc., and to legitimate the general
status quo in health-care, which is characterized by free-
enterprise providers and a medical monopoly over diagno-
sis and treatment.

However, organizations providing and financing health-
care have been hampered in their ability to fully introduce these socio-political changes by two external forces.
The first force is the growing concern of monopoly capital
as a whole with both the escalating cost of health-care
for its workers and the preservation of private enterprise in health-care. The second force comes from workers and consumers. They, like employers, are becoming
more and more angry at the high cost of health-care.
Workers and consumers are also getting angry at the inhu-
manity and limited efficacy of that care, and at their
inability to influence health-care institutions. These
two forces mean that there are many "eddies" running
counter to the main "stream" that was described in the
previous paragraph. In particular, Marxists predict that
medical ideologies will display an acceptance of large-
scale, high-technology settings of care, but will also
seek to legitimate the continuing control of those settings by physicians (as an "updated" version of the
petty-commodity mode) (McKinlay, unpublished: Navarro,
1976, 1978; Rodberg and Stevenson, 1977).[9]

---

[9]Rodberg and Stevenson (1977) term the current mode of
production in health-care the capitalist mode. This is a
misnomer, since the petty-commodity mode is also capitalist. At present, monopoly capital appears to be more
anxious about health-care cost-containment and about
general legitimation of the capitalist form of health-
care, than about some of the other functions that health-
care performs for monopoly capital, such as providing
investment outlets (Rodberg and Stevenson, 1977). An
additional cause of worker/consumer discontent that is

A third influential perspective on the medical profession is that of Eliot Freidson. Freidson makes two main points. First, physicians' behavior is influenced more by their immediate work settings and their operating norms than by the general norms and scientific knowledge they have internalized. Second, the typical work setting of contemporary doctors is, according to Freidson, one where doctors have been granted autonomy by some elite in the society. When we apply these two postulates to the analysis of ideological change in medicine, we encounter serious problems: unlike the Parsonian and Marxist approaches, Friedson's is primarily static; and it is unclear how the medical profession is granted autonomy by the state (McKinlay, 1977). Still, Freidson would probably argue that changes in the microstructures of work settings, and in the operative norms of those settings, lead to changes in the perceived crucial interests which doctors feel they must defend, and hence to changes in the nature of their ideological statements. Unlike Marxists, Freidson believes there has been no major reduction in physicians' autonomy since about 1960. Freidson would also presumably argue that doctors still see their ideological task as the defense of their autonomy. (Freidson, 1970a, 1970b, 1975).[10]

Parsons, Marx and Freidson: Empirical Indicators.

It is evident that Parsons and the Marxists offer highly complex explanations of trends in medical ideologies, and in the health-care system as a whole. If we try to test the two explanations, we will not find it easy to operationalize the major variables and the relationships between those variables. However, we suggest

---

somewhat relevant is capital's increasingly salient role in causing workplace hazards and pollution. These popular sentiments appear to have less impact on demands regarding terminal care than do worker/consumer anger over health-care services.

[10]We should mention briefly the current popular view that physicians are the primary cause of the expansion of biomedical technology and of medical definitions of social and personal problems (Illich, 1976; cf. Navarro, 1976: 103-34). While exponents of this view disagree with Parsonians and with Freidson on many points, they do agree on the basic claim that the medical profession is autonomous. The Parsonian perspective is also unable to predict at least one trend in the dependent variable, namely the growing emphasis in the JCD on doctors' collaboration with their "team-mates". Parsonians--who are much more explicit about terminal-care ideologies than Marxists-- claim that doctors still claim exclusive authority over every patient's treatment (Parsons et al., 1973).

the following types of evidence are the most important. We will focus on the various independent variables (not the dependent variable of medical ideologies of terminal care).

For a Parsonian, the first type of data concerns research and development of major new technologies affecting doctors' power over death. Especially important is research and development that takes place in medical schools and hospitals, rather than in private industry or government agencies, since the former stems most directly from the knowledge and values of physicians themselves. Second, evidence would be sought of changes in the public's general attitudes towards scientific and rational approaches to human problems--which would indicate the types of broad cultural pressures to which physicians have to respond in advancing medical technologies. Third, the general normative statements and practices of the medical profession would receive attention, regarding such issues as whether doctors have the right to define and manage all aspects of health, ethical standards for health-care workers and patients, and the rights of different social strata to health services (cf. Parsons et al., 1973: 20-21). Finally, these statements would be linked to changing public attitudes on these matters, and to demands by legitimate public leaders (clergypersons, lawyers, scientists, etc.) that the medical profession clarify or change its stance in these areas. We should add that data on all these four topics should reflect not only formal organizational behaviour and official statements, but also informal behaviour and unofficial opinions.

A Marxist might document the changing mode of production of health care by describing the growing use in different care settings of expensive high technology equipment such as CAT scanners. Regarding the accompanying social and political changes we have discussed, the choice of indicators is relatively easy. For instance, we need to know the changing proportion of terminal care actually given in hospitals as compared with patients' homes. (Nursing homes are an important setting of terminal care. They should probably be classified as employing a petty-commodity mode of production in most cases). In addition, we would need to know whether leading medical schools and large hospitals are increasingly often represented on federal policy-making committees, and on drug-company boards of directors. We would also look at the frequency with which leading business associations, labor unions, and consumer groups demand that health-care cost inflation be curtailed.

However, it is not easy to show the relative severity of the various contradictions that accompany the general trend. Possible evidence for contradictions includes the changing volume and content of public self-justifications by leading hospitals, insurance companies, etc.; and the extent to which physicians engage in public debates on major health-care issues (when collecting these data, we should also examine the protagonists' specialties and institutional affiliations).

As we have indicated, Freidson (unlike both Parsons and the Marxists) has not articulated an explicit model of ideological change in medicine. But he would probably look especially at developments such as the changing use of attending hospital physicians as opposed to office-based solo practitioners, and at trends in the complexity and size of the "teams" that actually care for patients. Regarding normative changes at the workplace, Freidson would be particularly interested in the changing extent to which doctors were expected to respond to the needs--even orders--of the team as a whole, of the organizations where they worked, and of their professional associations.

We should now move on to some empirical data. Before doing so, we should mention that we present no data to test the usefulness of Freidson's perspective. We do this for two reasons. First, Freidson does not have a systematic theory of ideological change. Second, some of the general causal factors mentioned by Freidson are similar to some of those mentioned by the Parsonians, while others of Freidson's factors overlap with the Marxists'. Accordingly, in a preliminary analysis like this one, where we cannot be sure about even the hypothetical relationships between the variables, it is more appropriate to test two perspectives--the Marxist and the Parsonian--that are, roughly speaking, mutually exclusive.

We have only been able to collect readily-available published data that bear on our two perspectives. We have chosen data that unambiguously reflect either the Parsonian or the Marxist approach, but not both. Unfortunately, such data are too crude to permit an analysis of possible dialectic processes. In interpreting the various time-series presented below, we follow the elementary rule that if a change in an independent variable happened after a change in the dependent variable, that independent variable does not operate as a cause.

Evidence for a Parsonian Explanation

If the Parsonian explanation of medical ideologies is correct, we should find that medical schools--which are among the main institutions for the socialization of professional norms--formally expressed a concern with the care of the dying before the profession as a whole. However, the evidence suggests that the nation's medical schools typically followed rather than led the general profession on terminal-care issues. According to Cumulated Index Medicus, it was not until 1970 that any medical-education journal mentioned the care of the dying, or any medical school offered formal courses on this topic. (Dickinson, 1976; Liston, 1973, 1975).

Another implication of the Parsonian perspective is that the most prestigious medical journals will be concerned with terminal-care issues, before "rank-and-file" medical journals. This, it is held, is because the leaders of the profession feel duty-bound to be the first physicians to seriously discuss and disseminate new knowledge and values. Yet in the very prestigious New England Journal of Medicine there was not (according to Cumulated Index Medicus) a single article, editorial or letter on terminal care until 1968, i.e., after the attainment of a generally-higher level of concern with the dying in the general medical literature.[11] Similarly, in the JCD normative themes usually changed only in 1969,[12] and the number of statements on terminal care only increased in 1969[13] (see Section II).

However, calls in the JCD for closer cooperation with colleagues, and for respect for the right to die, are consistent with the Parsonian view that in the sixties the medical profession took a more relativistic view of terminal-care ethics. But even granting this, we must still mention as evidence against the Parsonian perspective the fact that the new, more relativistic ethic was not expressed in the JCD until 1969, i.e., after interest in terminal care markedly escalated in less prestigious journals.

Evidence for a Marxist Explanation

One important indicator of the changing mode of production in health-care is the diffusion of complex biomedical technologies in hospitals. Russell (1976) has shown that between 1953 and 1974, the proportion of middle-sized hospitals possessing diagnostic radio-isotope equipment, electro-encephalograph machines, and cobalt therapy equipment--all techniques frequently used in the treatment of terminal diseases--have grown steadily, but without any sudden spurts.[14]

---

[11]A detailed content analysis of statements on terminal care in the New England Journal of Medicine is undertaken in MacDougall and Ost, unpublished.

[12]An exception is Hinton (1964).

[13]This is particularly true if we bear in mind that in 1963, there were three articles on terminal care--exceptionally large number--in the JCD.

[14]The proportion of hospitals using radium and x-ray therapy facilities actually fell after the early 1960s, because those technologies became obsolete (Russell, 1976: 566). Russell's data on cobalt and radium therapy equipment only cover the period 1965-74.

Turning to the important socio-political concomitants of the changed mode of production, let us first examine the penetration of terminal-care settings by corporate capital. An indicator of this penetration is the extent to which terminal-care goods and services are bought from profit-making corporations. A rough estimate of such purchases can be made on the basis of Stevenson's (1976) data on corporate sales to the whole health-care system. In Table 7.3, we have selected those goods and services mentioned by Stevenson that are most frequently used in the treatment of dying patients. The figures show large absolute increases in corporate sales, but no growth in such sales relative to all terminal-care-related expenditures. This trend is consistent with the gradual diffusion of high-technology equipment in hospitals, which we noted in the preceding paragraph--a diffusion than can also be used to measure corporate penetration of terminal care. Returning to Stevenson's data, we also find that in almost all sectors, the most rapid expansion in profit-making corporations' activity occurred during the years 1967-1972. This was after the growth in expressions of ideological concern about the dying in the medical literature. It is interesting that we do not find in the JCD any statement that the medical profession should defend health-care corporations.

An indicator of the growing influence of hospital and other administrators' power over doctors is that the proportion of physicians who are salaried employees has grown somewhat between 1963 and 1973. (McKinlay, unpublished).

Moreover, according to the Marxist position, doctors are increasingly financed-but also regulated-by the state. A rough measure of this trend is the preparation of health care expenditures by the aged that are met by government programs. This proportion suddenly doubled after the introduction of Medicare and Medicaid in 1966, and thereafter remained at about 60 percent.[15] This spurt in governmental activity occurred at just the time when professional medical interest in terminal care increased markedly, as shown in Section II. (Cooper and Worthington, 1973a, 1973b; Mueller and Gibson, 1976).

Several of the thematic changes in the JCD that we traced in Section II may be seen as justification of the changes in doctors' typical social relations of production

---

[15]There appears to be no information on the proportion of the elderly's health-care expenditures paid for by the government before 1966. But we know that for all age-groups, the proportion of health-care expenditures paid by the government rose sharply after 1966, from a little over 20 percent between 1950 and 1965, to about 35 percent in the late 1960s (Cooper and Worthington, 1973a).

TABLE 7.3
Expenditures by Profit-Making Organizations of Terminal-Care Related Goods and Services, 1962-75

Year	On Drugs and Sundries		On Eyeglasses And Appliances		Hospitals--Profit-Making Component**		Nursing Homes--Profit-Making Component**		All Profit-Making Organizations		All Relevant Health-Care Expenditures ($ Million)*	
	Increase	Share of all relevant exp's	Increase	Share....	Increase	Share....	Increase	Share....	Increase	Share....	Expenditures	Increase
1962		17.1%		3.9%		16.2%		2.1%		39.4%	23696	
1962-67	33.8%		66.7%		37.6%		202.8%		56.9%			61.9%
1967		14.3%		3.9%		16.0%		4.0%		38.2%	38361	
1967-72	50.3%		24.0%		95.9%		200.5%		83.3%			83.8%
1972		11.7%		2.7%		17.1%		6.5%		37.9%	70503	
1972-75	28.7%		22.5%		46.4%		56.4%		40.9%			38.0%
1975		10.9%		2.4%		18.1%		7.3%		38.7%	97293	

Table 7.3 cont'd.

Source: Stevenson, 1976: 2-3

*The sum of: 1) drugs and sundries, 2) eyeglasses and
appliances, 3) hospitals, 4) physicians' services, 5)
other professional services, and 6) expenses for prepayment and administration. The expenditures omitted--
dentists' services, government public health, research,
construction, and other health services--constituted a
slowly-declining proportion of all health-care expenditures (17.9% in 1975).
**The sum of: 1) all expenditures by profit-making
hospitals or nursing homes, and 2) for non-profit hospitals or nursing homes, expenditures on food, supplies,
drugs, etc.

For instance, there were in the late 1960s and 1970s
increasingly frequent calls for cooperation among professionals in terminal-care teams, and members of those
teams include such state employees as social workers.
Yet in these statements, the doctors' position as the
most powerful stratum in health-care delivery institutions is frequently justified.[16]
Perhaps too, the growing insistence in the medical
literature on honesty towards patients reflects an ero-
sion of physicians' absolute authority over patient care,
and also reflects doctors' need to work in somewhat egal-
itarian teams. For in a setting of team care, patients
are probably more likely to learn the truth from non-
physician professionals than if the doctor were the
undisputed boss. In that event, doctors' prestige is
probably better maintained if they are the first professionals to level with patients. Moreover, a doctor
who is honest may avoid a malpractice suit. These
hypotheses require further research.

CONCLUSIONS

Summary of Findings

We found in Section II that the number of articles,
editorials and letters on the norms of terminal care in
the medical literature was larger after 1967, both in all
medical journals and in the JCD. We also found that in

---

[16]A good example of this ideological stance is found in
the widely discussed guidelines proposed at the very
prestigious Massachusetts General Hospital in 1976, and
published in the New England Journal of Medicine.
(Critical Care Committee, 1976.)

the late sixties and seventies--but not before--doctors were urged to be truthful with dying patients, and to cooperate more closely with other members of the terminal-care team.

In Section III we attempt a preliminary explanation of these findings. We assessed the relative merits of the Parsonian and Marxist perspectives by examining some readily available time-series data. These data do not support the Parsonian perspective. But they are consistent with a Marxist perspective, to the extent that simultaneous with the rise in medical interest in terminal care, there was an increase in the medical profession's employment on salary, and in state funding of terminal care. These changes are prima facie consistent with the argument that doctors have become increasingly involved in "large-scale, high technology" mode and relations of production.

Suggestions for Further Research

Further research is clearly needed, not only to enlarge the data-base on the nature of medical ideologies, but also to refine and augment the indicators of possible causes of those ideologies. Specific variables to be studied have been discussed in Section III. Parsonians, Marxists and Freidsonians would all do well to reanalyze ethnographies of medical schools, hospitals and other institutions where health-care is delivered and health-care workers trained. Since the studies were conducted at a different time, data from them, where comparable, constitute a rough time-series (see for example, Becker et al., 1961; Fox, 1959; Gubrium, 1975; Quint, 1967; Millman, 1976; Sudnow, 1967). For a Parsonian, a useful source of data would be general normative and technical statements in both medical and popular mass media, attitude surveys of both the public and professionals, and community studies (as indicators of popular values and beliefs). For a Marxist, additional information could be found in "political-economy" type histories of relevant technologies, and of major agencies engaged in health-care services, research and funding;[17] in time-series of employment in specialized occupations and work settings; and in the occupations and work settings; and in the occupational and institutional backgrounds of those publicly expressing different points of view.

It would be of great interest to assess the relative

---

[17]The studies by Feder (1977) and Strickland (1972) are good examples of recent work on specific agencies. Those by Russell (1976) and Stevenson (1976) are good starting points for an analysis of aggregate time-series data.

explanatory power of a Marxist and a Freidsonian perspective, since Freidson is very influential among medical sociologists today. A conclusive test of the two perspectives would require a careful examination of which independent variables applied only to one perspective, and which applied to both perspectives. Changes in doctors' work settings are probably relevant to both perspectives, while changes in state activities and in worker or consumer demands can only be used to test a Marxist explanation.[18]

Researches such as these will help us understand more clearly not only the changing nature of terminal care, but also the general situation of the whole medical profession. This situation is obviously undergoing major changes, but those changes are still poorly understood.

REFERENCES

Becker, Howard S., Blanche Geer, Everett Hughes and Anselm Strauss
    1961   Boys in White. Chicago: University of Chicago Press.
Blishen, Bernard R.
    1969   Doctors and Doctrine: The Ideology of Medical Care in Canada. Toronto: University of Toronto Press.
Conner, J.F., F.B. Devitt and H.J. Switkes
    1955   "A hospital unit for the care of the patient with long-term illness: the intermediate service." Journal of Chronic Diseases 2: 167-179.
Cooper, Barbara S. and Nancy L. Worthington
    1975a   "Age differences in medical care spending, fiscal year 1972." Social Security Bulletin 36: 3-15.
    1973b   "National Health Expenditures." Social Security Bulletin 36: 3-19, 40.
Crane, Diana
    1975   The Sanctity of Social Life. New York: Russell Sage Foundation.

---

[18]The differences between a Marxist and a Freidsonian explanation are explored in detail in MacDougall and Ost, unpublished. Many of Friedson's concepts and generalizations have strongly influenced Marxist analyses of health care. Freidson's approach also overlaps with Parsons' in Freidson's emphasis on internalized norms as a factor influencing doctors' behavior. However, for Parsons, those norms are general while for Freidson they are situational.

Critical Care Committee
    1976   "Optimum care for hopelessly ill patients."
            New England Journal of Medicine 195: 364-66.
Dickinson, George E.
    1976   "Death Education in U.S. Medical Schools."
            Journal of Medical Education 51: 134-36.
Feder, Judith M.
    1977   Medicare: The Politics of Federal Hospital
            Insurance. Lexington, Mass.: Heath.
Fox, Renee C.
    1959   Experiment Perilous: Physicians and Patients
            Facing the Unknown. Glencoe, Ill.: The Free
            Press.
Freidson,Eliot
    1970a   Profession of Medicine. New York: Dodd Mead.
    1970b   Professional Dominance. Chicago: Aldine.
    1975   Doctoring Together: A Study of Professional
            Social Control. New York: Elsevier.
Gubrium, Jaber F.
    1975   Living and Dying at Murray Manor. New York:
            St. Martin's
Hinton, John M.
    1964   "Editorial: Problems in the Care of the
            Dying." Journal of Chronic Diseased 17:
            203-204.
Illich, Ivan
    1976   Medical Nemesis: The Expropriation of
            Health. New York: Random House.
Iszak, F.C., J. Engel and J.H. Medalie
    1973   "Comprehensive Rehabilitation of the Patient
            with Cancer." Journal of Chronic Diseases
            27: 201-212.
Lasagna, Louis
    1969   "Editorial: The Doctor and the Dying
            Patient." Journal of Chronic Diseases 22:
            67-69.
Life-in-Death
    1957   "Life-in-Death."   New England Journal of
            Medicine 256: 760-61.
Liston, Edward H.
    1973   "Education on Death and Dying: A Survey of
            American Medical Schools." Journal of Medical
            Education 48: 577-78.
    1975   "Education on Death and Dying: A Neglected
            Area in the Medical Curriculum."   Omega 6:
            193-98.
MacDougall, John and John Ost
    Unpub. "Doctors, Death and Dying: Some Ideological
            Trends."
MacDougall, John and Marilyn M. Rawnsley
    1978   "Power, Professionals and New Ways of Dying."
            Paper presented at the Annual Meeting of the
            American Sociological Association.

McKinlay, John B.
    1977   "The business of good doctoring or doctoring as good business: Reflections on Freidson's View of the Medical Game." International Journal of Health Services 7: 459-83.
    Unpub. "Towards the Proletarianization of Physicians."

Merton, Robert K., George C. Reeder and Patricia L. Kendall, eds.,
    1957   The Student Physician. Cambridge: Harvard University Press.

Millman, Marcia
    1976   The Unkindest Cut: Life in the Backrooms of Medicine. New York: Morrow.

Mueller, Marjorie S. and Richard K. Gibson
    1976   "Age Differencs in Health Care Spending, Fiscal Year 1975." Social Security Bulletin 39: 18-31.

Okun, Donald
    1961   "What to Tell Cancer Patients: A Study of Medical Attitudes." Journal of the American Medical Association 175: 1120-28.

Navarro, Vicente
    1976   Medicine Under Capitalism. New York: Prodist.
    1978   "The Crisis of the Western System of Medicine in Contemporary Capitalism." International Journal of Health Services 8: 179-211.

Newell, R.R.
    1958   "What Should We Tell the Patient?" Journal of Chronic Diseases 7: 52-57.

Parsons, Talcott
    1972   "Definitions of Health and Illness in the Light of American Values." Pp. 107-27 in E. Gartly Jaco, (ed.), Patients, Physicians and Illness, second ed. New York: The Free Press.

Parsons, Talcott, Renee C. Fox and Victor Lidz
    1973   "The Gift of Life and Its Reciprocation." Pp. 1-49 in Arien Mack (ed.), Death in American Experience. New York: Schocken.

Parsons, Talcott, and Victor Lidz.
    1967   "Death in American Society." Pp. 133-70 in Edwin S. Schneidman (ed.), Essays in Self-Destruction. New York: Science House.

Quint, Jeanne C.
    1967   The Nurse and the Dying Patient. New York: Macmillan.

Rodberg, Leonard and Gelvin Stevenson
    1977   "The Health Care Industry in Advanced Capitalism." Review of Radical Political Economics 9: 104-14.

Russell, Louise B.
    1976   "The Diffusion of New Hospital Technologies
            in the United States." International Journal
            of Health Services 6: 557-580.
Schulz, Ronald and David Aderman
    1976   "How the Medical Staff Copes with Dying
            Patients." Omega 7: 11-21.
Senescu, Richard A.
    1963   "The Development of Emotional Complication in
            the Patient with Cancer." Journal of Chronic
            Diseases 16: 825-832.
Stevenson, Gelvin
    1976   "Profits in Medicine." Health-PAC Bulletin 72:
            2-16.
Strickland, Stephen P.
    1972   Politics, Science and Dread Disease: A Short
            History of United States Medical Research
            Policy. Cambridge: Harvard University Press.
Sudnow, David
    1967   Passing on: The Social Organization of
            Dying. Englewood Cliffs, N.J.: Prentice-Hall.
Theologides, Athanasios
    1971   "Editorial: Oncology Service in a Teaching
            Hospital." Journal of Chronic Diseases 23:
            601-604.
Wallace, Anthony F.C.
    1956   "Revitalization   Movements."   American
            Anthropologist 58.
Waterman, Barbara and Howard Waitzkin
    Unpub. "Ideology and Social Control in the Doctor-
            Patient Relationship."

8

The Triumph of Chiropractic– and Then What?

Walter I. Wardwell   University of Connecticut

The evolution of chiropractic from a marginal health profession to the strongest and most popular alternative to orthodox medicine in the United States is examined and compared with osteopathy and naturopathy. Evidence is offered that 1974 was the landmark year for recognition of chiropractors (e.g., accreditation of colleges, reimbursement for services under Medicare) and relaxation of the American Medical Association's policy of active and overt opposition (e.g., elimination from its code of ethics of the tabu on professional association. The public policy question of the future status of chiropractors is raised and alternatives considered. It is concluded that the most likely outcome, as well as the best for all concerned, is for chiropractic to evolve to a "limited medical" professional status comparable to that of dentistry, podiatry, optometry, and psychology.

Of all the alternative forms of health delivery in the United States at the present time, chiropractors and chiropractic treatment are without doubt the most prominent example. Ever since 1895 when Daniel David Palmer gave his first "adjustment" in Davenport, Iowa, chiropractic has been the alternative most offensive to the medical establishment, perhaps precisely because it has been so successful. Its survival is a historical fact that cannot be swept under the rug by pretending that it is merely passing fad, a popular fancy that will go away as soon as lay people have been properly informed by expert medical opinion. Since World War II chiropractic has become stronger rather than weaker, and it certainly shows no sign of disappearing.

Chiropractors maintain, of course, that the reason for chiropractic's survival are to be found in its effectiveness as a system of therapy. Organized medicine, on the other hand, has viewed chiropractic as an unscientific cult, and chiropractors as, at best, misguided and unqualified, or as out-and-out quacks. As a result, no objective evaluation of chiropractic in the form of a clinical trial has ever been conducted, although an effort to complete such an evaluation is being made in Toronto; so far no results are available.

Pending final judgement by medical historians as to the reasons why chiropractic has survived despite the mightiest efforts of organized medicine to eliminate it, comparison with the histories of osteopathy and naturopathy offers some insight into the alternatives that could have befallen chiropractic in the past and still might occur in the future. The evolution of osteopathy to near-fusion with medicine and the near-demise of naturopathy illumine the possibilities for chiropractic.

OSTEOPATHY

Andrew Taylor Still created osteopathy at least twenty years before chiropractic appeared although he did not found his college until 1892. A frontier medical doctor, his objective was to reform medicine rather than to supplant it, as is clear from the 1894 charter of his American School of Osteopathy (later the Kirksville College of Osteopathy) in Kirksville, Missouri, which stated, in part:

> ...to establish a college of osteopathy, the design of which is to improve our present system of surgery, obstetrics and treatment of diseases generally, and place the same on a more rational and scientific basis, and to impart information to the medical profession and to grant and confer such honors and degrees as are usually granted and conferred by reputable medical colleges (Northup, 1972).

Despite Still's original principles that the body is its own laboratory and that health lies in maintaining the structural integrity of the body through osteopathic manipulation, and despite Still's hostility to drugs and surgery, osteopathic colleges, unlike chiropractic colleges, have always taught the full range of medical subjects, including surgery and materia-medica, and thus their curricula have always paralleled the scope, if not the quality, of medical schools.

However, the American Medical Association (AMA) always considered osteopathy sectarian medicine. In Morris Fishbein's (1925) famous phrase osteopathy was "essentially a method of entering the practice of medicine" by the backdoor. The AMA's lingering hostility toward osteopathy was evident in its 1961 decision to permit its constituent state medical societies to make the determination whether to accept individual osteopaths as professional equals:

> The test should be: Does the individual doctor of
> osteopathy practice osteopathy or does he in fact
> practice a method of healing founded on a scientific
> basis? (Osteopathy..., 1961).

The present strategy of the AMA, in contrast to its
continued opposition to chiropractic, clearly is to bring
osteopathy within the medical fold by recognizing
osteopaths as fully qualified physicians, by eliminating
the few remaining legal restrictions on osteopaths' scope
of practice, and by accepting graduates of osteopathic
colleges into residencies and as candidates for medical
board certification. The AMA's most striking success in
this new strategy was to persuade the California College
of Osteopathic Physicians and Surgeons (by a one-vote
majority of its board!) to become the University of
California College of Medicine, Irvine, and the state
osteopathic and medical societies to merge. Since then
the American Osteopathic Association (AOA) has reacted
strongly to the threat of being absorbed into medicine
and has added nine new osteopathic colleges to the five
then remaining. Present-day osteopathic colleges are
essentially medical schools with one added subject in the
curriculm - OMT (osteopathic manipulative treatment); and
most osteopathic physicians (as they now prefer to be
called), especially the more recent graduates, practice
as medical doctors.

As osteopathy merges into the medical mainstream, it
appears to be repeating the history of homeopathy, which
for two thirds of the nineteenth century was a separate
"school" of medicine based on the distinctive therapeutic
doctrines of "similars" and "infinitessimals." With
their own schools and hospitals, homeopaths vied for
popular favor with orthodox physicians, whom they called
"allopaths", a term that has stuck. (In 1908, according
to Kaufman (1971:167), graduates of homeopathic colleges
performed better on state licensing examinations than
did the graduates of allopathic colleges.) Toward the
end of the nineteenth century, however, contention between homeopaths and allopaths waned as their modes of
practice became less differentiated and as organized
medicine perceived more serious threats from osteopathy
and chiropractic. Homeopathic colleges like Hahnemann
(named for the founder of homeopathy) and Boston
University eventually became conventional medical schools
producing graduates who consider themselver orthodox physicians. The same process seems to be at work with
osteopathy.

NATUROPATHY

Briefer comments can be made about naturopathy, which for many years struggled for preeminence with chiropractic. It is a form of drugless healing that incorporates a variety of "natural" treatment modalities such as heat, light, water, vitamin and food supplements, and physical therapy in addition to spinal manipulation. Although Twaddle and Hessler (1977:166) suggest that there is a link between homeopathy and naturopathy, it probably does not involve direct lineage but merely naturopathic interest in certain homeopathic remedies. With such a positively-toned name, "naturopathy" ought to have carried greater public appeal, as a label, than the awkward neologism "chiropractic," especially during recent years when there has been so much interest in natural foods, natural living exercise, avoiding food additives and drugs, etc. In earlier years the "mixer" wing of the chiropractic colleges often offered courses in naturopathy along with chiropractic or offered two separate programs and degrees (D.C. and N.D.). Three of the currently accredited chiropractic colleges did so as late as 1948. Nevertheless, naturopathy seems to be losing its struggle to survive. With only one or two very small schools remaining, and some of the states that formerly licensed them no longer doing so, very few new graduates are entering the field.

Relatively few people have ever heard of naturopathy, probably because drugless healing has been nearly preempted by chiropractic. I earlier advanced two main reasons to explain why chiropractic came to dominate drugless healing at the expense of naturopathy (Wardwell, 1978). One is that naturopathy did not have a distinctive therapeutic focus as chiropractic did with its theory of spinal subluxations, but involved a miscellaneous collection of natural remedies. The other reason is probably more important. It is that naturopathy lacked a charismatic leader like B.J. Palmer (the son of the founder) around whom or in opposition to whom chiropractors could rally. So despite the attractiveness of the word "naturopathy", it has lost out to chiropractic, with the result that some chiropractors who also possess an N.D. degree no longer display it.

CHIROPRACTIC'S SURVIVAL

Unlike osteopathy, whose creator never thought of himself as other than a medical doctor with an improved therapeutic philosophy, chiropractic was begun by an outsider to the medical profession. For ten years prior to his "discovery" of chiropractic, Daniel David Palmer had been a magnetic healer, before that a grocer and fish dealer. Although allegedly chiropractic was "stolen"

from osteopathy (Bayer, 1945), Palmer advanced a somewhat
different theory of illness and therapy. He developed
the concept of the <u>subluxation</u> (misalignment) of vertebrae
as interfering with neural transmission to vital organs,
thus causing disease, which requires correction through
"adjustment" of the misaligned vertebrae, thus restoring
normal functioning. (The osteopathic term for subluxa-
tion is "osteopathic lesion," while medical doctors
prefer the term "joint disfunction.") (Northup, 1972;
Mennell, 1975). Although a recent article (Gibbons,
1979) documents early interest in chiropractic and collaboration by orthodox physicians, organized medicine con-
demned the medical heresy outright. Palmer's son, "B.J.",
further widened the gap between them by arguing that
chiropractic is philosophically the exact opposite of
medicine:

> The dividing line is sharply drawn - anything given,
> applied to, or prescribed from outside-in, below-up,
> comes within the principle and practice of medicine.
> None of this does chiropractic do! Our principle is
> opposite, antipodal, the reverse, for everything
> within the chiropractic philosophy, science and art
> works from above-down, inside-out. Anything and
> everything outside that scope is medicine, whether
> you like it or not (Palmer, 1958).

Palmer's strategy enabled him to argue that chiropractic
is a separate and distinct science and therefore should
have separate schools, licensing laws, and examining
boards. Although he naturally attributed chiropractic's
success to its superior efficacy, it was certainly due in
part to his own charismatic leadership that chiropractic
survived as a separate and distinct health profession.
Rejected by medicine and osteopathy, B.J. Palmer made a
virtue out of necessity. He trained thousands of
chiropractors, sold them millions of tracts for distribution to patients, persuaded legislatures to establish
separate laws and licensing boards, and successfully
defended accused chiropractors in court. Despite the
many rifts within the profession that his strong per-
sonality caused, he inspired his followers to heal the
sick, to fight for their profession, and always to send
him more students. (The Palmer School in 1922 had 3100
students enrolled). He wanted chiropractic "pure,
straight and unadulterated", and his followers were
called "straights." He opposed mixing chiropractic with
medicine, osteopathy, naturopathy, or physiotherapy, and
called chiropractors who did so "mixers." Such a mono-
causal theory of illness and treatment caused the AMA to
label chiropractic a "cult" although more than half of
all chiropractors have been mixers to some degree. But
without B.J. Palmer chiropractic probably would not have

survived at all.

B.J. Palmer also made it unlikely that chiropractic will ever follow the path of osteopathy toward medical orthodoxy. The social and professional cleavages between medicine and chiropractic remain too great. He also ensured that chiropractic would not become identified with naturopathy, which could easily have happened in view of the fact that some chiropractic colleges also offered naturopathic courses and degrees. It is probably best to conceive the evolution of chiropractic as a social movement, for it originated during a period of dissatisfaction with medical orthodoxy, was led by a charismatic leader who inspired awe and devotion, was supported by followers whose loyalty Palmer reinforced by frequent reunions, hortative writings, and speeches, and prospered in the favorable legal and political environment that he created. Although it also required satisfied patients, a major factor in the success of the movement was the professional identity and solidarity of Palmer's followers in his "straight" International Chiropractors Association or of his opponents in the "mixer" American Chiropractic Association.

What kinds of patients did chiropractic attract? Predictably, many came out of desperation that medicine had not helped them - as one chiropractor bemoaned: "after they have exhausted medical science and their money." And many were helped. Some patients perceived chiropractors as another kind of medical specialist. The contrary view of organized medicine is that most of the benefits that patients receive from chiropractic are psychological - either the patient had an imaginary illness or he only imagined that he was cured.

There is a paucity of good data concerning the educational or socioeconomic levels of chiropractic patients. However, a recent household survey (Advancedata, 1978) revealed that high users of chiropractic were more likely to be white than black, middle-aged rather than young or aged, middle income rather than low or high income. While there is some evidence that chiropractic has attracted more patients in rural than in urban areas (McCorkle, 1961), the same is probably also true of osteopathy; the explanation could be simply that both originated in the basically rural areas of the American mid-West.

CHIROPRACTIC'S TRIUMPH

Although the chiropractic profession seemed most appropriately characterized as "marginal" when I introduced that term nearly thirty years ago (Wardwell, 1951), its status has greatly improved since then. In 1974, four events occurred signalling that chiropractic has attained the status of an established profession in the

United States. First, the only remaining state that had not previously licensed chiropractors (Louisiana) passed legislation to do so. Second, the United States Office of Education recognized officially the Chiropractic Association as the accrediting agency for chiropractic colleges. Third, the United States Congress began payments for chiropractors' services under the Medicare program, and fourth, the Congress directed that $2,000,000 be used to study the research status of chiropractic.

The significance of the last item requires elucidation. It was decided that the National Institutes of Health should hold a Workshop to provide a basis for determining subsequent steps. Designated as Chairman was the Associate Director of the National Institute of Neurological and Communicative Disorders and Stroke, an osteopath, who was assigned a Workshop Planning Committee of leading medical scientists, osteopaths, and chiropractors to assist him. It was the first major effort ever by an interdisciplinary group of distinguised researchers and clinicians to examine spinal manipulative therapy in a scientific conclave. Since the topic of the Workshop became the scientific status of <u>spinal manipulative therapy</u> rather than the scientific status of <u>chiropractic</u>, the onus became shifted partly away from chiropractors onto osteopaths and those medical doctors who use spinal manipulative therapy. The latter have organized themselves into a small group called the North American Academy of Manipulative Medicine. Naturally those osteopaths and MD's who use spinal manipulative therapy agree with chiropractors that there is a scientific basis for it. The resulting publication containing the papers presented at the workshop (Goldstein, 1975) was supportive of spinal manipulative therapy although a few of the medical doctors who participated were clearly hostile to it. The majority consensus was that the reasons why spinal manipulative therapy is effective are not well understood and therefore more research is needed. Since then, the National Institutes of Health have made several grants of federal money to support such research, which several chiropractors have collaborated in.

The first truly objective study of chiropractors, which incidentally recommends their incorporation into the health delivery system in New Zealand, was recently published by an official Commission of Inquiry (1979).

Two other developments documenting the increased acceptance of chiropractors in the United States occurred in 1976. The first was a study authorized by Congress:

> to determine the average annual per student educational cost of providing educational programs which lead to a degree of doctor of chiropractic... The study shall also determine the current demand for

chiropractic services throughout the United States
and shall develop methodologies for determining if
current supply of chiropractors is sufficient to meet
this demand (Chiropractic Health Care, 1980).

The second was a major anti-trust court suit entered by
five chiropractors against the AMA, the American College
of Surgeons, the American College of Physicians, the
American Hospital Association, and the American
Osteopathic Association, plus seven other medical organizations and four individuals for having:

conspired to monopolize health care services in the
United States and conspired to unreasonably restrain
duly liscensed chiropractic doctors including the
plaintiffs herein from competing with medical doctors
in the delivery of health care services to the
general public in the United States, and moreover,
have been and are engaged in a combination and
conspiracy to first isolate and then eliminate the
chiropractic profession in the United States (Wilk, et
al., 1976).

In addition to monetary damages and injunctions for
relief, the plaintiffs ask for:

establishment and maintenance for ten years at
defendants' sole expense and at a cost to defendants
of no less than $1,000,000 per year, of an inter-
professional research institute controlled equally
by medical doctors and Doctors of Chiropractic for
promoting inter-professional research and educational
programs, and for developing a common lexicon.

In July 1979 the Attorney General of the State of New
York (Note: a third party) initiated a similar suit on
behalf of the State and of all its citizens against the
AMA, AOA, the Medical Society of the State of New York,
the American Hospital Association, nine other medical
organizations, and one individual. It is expected that
these and additional suits filed in other states will
take a long time to be settled.
    Although the official position of the AMA continues to
be that chiropractic is an unscientific cult, an immediate result of the anit-trust suits is that the AMA has
ceased its public efforts to oppose chiropractors and
to prevent its own members from interacting professionally
with them. In March 1977, the AMA's Judicial Council
announced the opinion that:

A physician may refer a patient for diagnostic or
therapeutic services to another physician, a limited
practitioner, or any other provider of health care

services permitted by law to furnish such services, whenever he believes that this may benefit the patient. As in the case of referrals to physician-specialists, referrals to limited practitioners should be based on their individual competence and ability to perform the services needed by the patient (American Medical News, 1977).

The AMA also eliminated its Committee on Quackery and its Bureau of Investigation, both of which had expended most of their money and energy over many years primarily against chiropractors.

The result of all these developments is that chiropractic is now securely established as the leading drugless healing profession alternative to medicine in the United States. With over 23,000 practitioners chiropractic is nearly 50 percent larger than osteopathy; of all the health-related professionals only medical doctors, dentists, nurses, and pharmacists outnumber chiropractors. Of the sixteen chiropractic colleges in the United States most are either accredited or working toward accreditation (which requires a minimum of two years of pre-professinal college credits plus a four-year college program covering, in addition to chiropractic theory and practice, the standard medical curriculum except for surgery and pharmacology). The majority of the states have upgraded their licensing requirements to six post-secondary years of schooling. All the chiropractic colleges have retained Ph.D.'s to teach in the basic science areas and are beginning to sponsor research, since that is what the accrediting requirements stipulate. However, all too little good research has been done under chiropractic sponsorship, and the chiropractic colleges are still weak.

FUTURE POSSIBILITIES

These developments make the future relationship between chiropractic and medicine problematic and raise important policy questions for public health officials and health planners. From being a marginal profession chiropractic now seems to be becoming a profession "parallel" to medicine. This term better characterizes the relationship that is developing between them as chiropractors become more acceptable, as chiropractic theories become subjects for which the National Institutes of Health make university research grants, as chiropractic colleges lengthen and strengthen their programs of instruction, and as the legal and professional status of chiropractors becomes more firmly established. But chiropractic is not likely to follow the evolution of osteopathy from a "parallel" status toward fusion with medicine. The opposition of organized medicine is still too strong, and the hostility of chiropractors is still too intense for this to happen.

Nor would chiropractors be willing to work under physician prescription, as physical therapists do. As autonomous practitioners, they would lose by becoming mere ancillaries to physicians, who, in any case, would not often prescribe chiropractic treatment. Worth noting, however, is that this resolution to the problem of what to do about chiropractic is precisely what President Carter proposed to Congress on September 25, 1979, in his National Health Insurance Plan, though later changed to allow chiropractors independent status.

Of course it could happen that physical therapists would themselves take up spinal manipulative therapy in a major way, which some physicians (e.g., James Cyriax, 1978) and physical therapists (e.g., Stanley Paris) have urged. This would no doubt be the solution preferred by organized medicine because physicians would retain control and could decide whether to delegate the therapy to an assistant (the physical therapist). Although both Cyriax and Paris conduct workshops on spinal manipulative therapy for physical therapists and urge them to take it up, that would not solve the problem of what to do about chiropractors.

If physical therapists were to take up spinal manipulative therapy but practice independent of physical prescription, they would become essentially chiropractors themselves, which not only is very unlikely to happen, but would create still another group of independent practitioners.

One of two other outcomes is more likely to occur. The first is the status quo ante, where chiropractors would remain as B.J. Palmer wanted, a "separate and distinct" healing profession independent of medicine, though marginal to it and in overall social standing. Conceivably it might evolve to a "parallel" profession to medicine if it continues to gain in professional, scientific, and social standing, but sociological evidence suggests that "separate but equal" relationships are inherently unstable: either they don't remain equal, or they don't remain separate.

The final alternative would be for chiropractors to become what is called a "limited medical" profession (Wardwell, 1979). Examples of these are dentistry, podiatry, optometry, and psychology. Each of these deals with a part of the psychobiological organism and uses a limited range of diagnostic and therapeutic techniques of modalities compared with those of the physician. And they all accept the basic medical explanations of illness and therapy as expounded by medical science. That is, they don't challenge them, as chiropractors do, or maintain alternative theories of health and illness. They also recognize the medical doctor as the authority over

systemic illnesses and conditions requiring treatment by
controlled drugs or major surgery. Like marginal or
parallel practitioners, limited practitioners are
"portals of entry" into the health care system in the
sense that patients usually come directly to them without
having first been diagnosed by a physician and referred
by him to them.

While such a limited practitioner status would not be
welcomed by some chiropractors, particularly the most
doctrinaire who feel that chiropractic is not so limited
in what it can accomplish and who want nothing to do with
orthodox medical practice, it would however reflect the
reality of the way many chiropractors now practice. Of
course it would require some compromise of the original
simplistic chiropractic philosophy of disease and its
treatment. But chiropractors have already enthusiasti-
cally incorporated into their theories the most sophisti-
cated scientific findings from the fields of neuro-
physiology and spinal biomechanics, because they are
seen as evidence of the validity of chiropractic principles. The main area of scientific dispute appears to
lie in the question of how removed from the spine itself
the effects of neural interference or irritation can
extend (e.g., to extremities, internal organs). Some of
the historic claims of chiropractic might have to be
given up, but a cost-benefit analysis should make this
alternative attractive.

The limited practitioner alternative offers advantages
both to chiropractors and to the health care system if
all parties--chiropractors, organized medicine, and public
health officials and health planners--recognize reality
and not remain confused by partisan claims. The reality
is that most recent chiropractic graduates are well
grounded in the basic medical sciences and understand
quite well both the limits of chiropractic and the benefits of those medical prodecures which exceed their own
legal and technological capabilities. The reality is
that chiropractors frequently refer patients to M.D.'s or
other providers for conditions beyond their scope of
practice, and that more and more M.D.'s are referring
patients to chiropractors, though usually for a narrow
range of neuro-musculoskeletal conditions and especially
if the patients do not respond well to medical treatments. Hence, many chiropractors already practice as
limited medical practitioners in that they restrict their
scope to practice to a fairly narrow range of conditions
that they believe they can help. Of course, legally they
must limit the range of techniques they employ, principally to spinal manipulation, though fairly often with
the addition of some of the other "drugless" non-surgical
modalities, e.g., physical therapy, dietary supplements,
occasional psychological counseling, etc. Perhaps
equally important is the fact that third-party payments

tend to be limited to a narrow interpretation of a chiropractor's scope of practice, both as regards conditions treated and modalities employed.

Were chiropractors to adopt the "limited practitioner" model, they would continue to practice independent of physicians but give up their former cultist claims that they use a completely different theory of health and illness and can treat nearly all illnesses better than physicians. Within a more narrowly defined scope of practice they would continue to decide which patients to treat and how to treat them using the rather limited repertoire of modalities at their command. In so doing, they would not differ greatly from dentists, podiatrists, optometrists, or psychologists, who, after all, have secured established and indeed prestigious places in our health care system.

So this is the answer to "what then?" in my opinion. If chiropractic, the leading alternative health care profession in the United States, does not fade away (and that seems unlikely), if it is not taken over by orthodox medicine (which seems equally unlikely), and if it continues on its present road toward higher standards of education and training, better scientific research, well established relationships with other health providers, and ready reimbursement for its services by third-part payors including the government, the most appropriate solution is for chiropractic to compromise its original principles and to become a limited medical profession. There are many pressures pushing chiropractors in that direction, and many advantages to be gained for chiropractors, for organized medicine, and for our health care system.

REFERENCES

Advancedata
    1978   Utilization of Selected Medical Practitioners: United States, 1974. Advancedata from Vital and Health Statistics of the National Center for Health Statistics, No. 24 (March 24, 1978). USPHS, DHEW.
American Medical News
    1977   March 21.
Bayer, Charles M.
    1945   Medicine Men and Men of Medicine. New York: Public Relations Bureau, The Medical Society of the State of New York.
Chiropractic Health Care: A National Study of Cost of Education, Service Utilization, Number of Practicing Doctors of Chiropractic, and Other Key Policy Issues.
    1980   Health Services Administration, U.S. Department of Health, Education, and Welfare. (To be published).

Commission of Inquiry
    1979   Chiropractic in New Zealand. Wellington, NZ:
            P.D. Hasselberg, Government Printer.
Cyriax, James
    1978   Textbook of Orthopaedic Medicine. Vol. I.
            Seventh edition. London: Bailliere Tindal.
Fishbein, Morris
    1925   The Medical Follies. New York: Boni and
            Liveright.
Gibbons, Russell W.
    1980   "Physician-Chiropractors: Medical Presence
            in the Evolution of Chiropractic." Bulletin
            of the History of Medicine (in press).
Goldstein, Murray (ed.)
    1975   The Research Status of Spinal Manipulative
            Therapy: A Workshop held at the National In-
            stitutes of Health, February 2-4, 1975. Na-
            tional Institute of Neurological and Communi-
            cative Disorders and Stroke Monograph No. 15,
            Department of Health, Education, and Welfare
            publication (NIH76-998).   Washington, D.C.
Kane, Robert L.
    1974   "Manipulating   the   Patient."   Lancet
            7870:1333-6.
Kaufman, Martin
    1971   Homeopathy in America: The Rise and Fall of
            a Medical Heresy. Baltimore: Johns Hopkins
            Press.
McCorkle, Thomas
    1961   "Chiropractic: A Deviant Theory of Disease
            and   Treatment   in   Contemporary   Western
            Culture."   Human Organization 20 (Spring):
            20-23.
Mennell, John McM.
    1975   "History   of   the   Development   of   Medical
            Manipulative Concepts; Medical Terminology."
            Pp. 53-58 in Murray Goldstein (ed.), The
            Research   Status   of   Spinal   Manipulative
            Therapy: A workshop held at the National
            Institutes of Health, February 2-4, 1975.
            National   Institute   of   Neurological   and
            Communicative Disorders and Stroke Monograph
            No. 15, Department of Health, Education, and
            Welfare publication (NIH76-998). Washington,
            D.C.
Northup, George W.
    1972   Osteopathic   Medicine: An   American
            Reformation.   Chicago: American Osteopathic
            Association.
Osteopathy: Special Report of the Judicial Council to
            the AMA House of Delegates.
    1961   Journal of the American Medical Association
            177 (Sept. 16):744-76.

Palmer, Bartlett Joseph
    1958   Shall Chiropractic Survive? Davenport, Iowa:
            Palmer School of Chiropractic.
Twaddle, Andrew C., and Richard M. Hessler
    1977   A Sociology of Health.   St. Louis: C.V.
            Mosby.
U.S. Congress
    1976   Public Law 94-484, Section 902(a).
Wardwell, Walter I.
    1951   Social Strain and Social Adjustment in the
            Marginal Role of the Chiropractor.   Ph.D.
            dissertation, Harvard University.
    1952   "A   Marginal   Professional   Role: The
            Chiropractor." Social Forces 30:339-48.
    1978   "Social   Factors   in   the   Survival   of
            Chiropractic: A   Comparative   View."
            Sociological Symposium 22 (Spring): 6-17.
    1979   "Limited   and   Marginal   Practitioners."
            Chapter in H.E. Freeman, S. Levine, and L.G.
            Reeder (eds.), Handbook of Medical Sociology.
            Third   Edition.   Englewood   Cliffs,   NJ:
            Prentice-Hall.
Wilk, Chester A., James W. Bryden, Patricia B. Arthur,
            Steven G. Lumsden, and Michael D. Pedigo
    1976   Complaint #76C3777 filed October 12 in the
            U.S. District Court for the Northern District
            of Illinois, Eastern Division.

9
The Good Life: Who's Practicing Healthy Life-Styles?

Ann S. Ford and W. Scott Ford
Florida State University

> The greatest current potential for improving the health of the American people is to be found in what they do or don't do to and for themselves.
>
> Victor Fuchs, Who Shall Live?

With the birth of scientific medicine in the late 1800s, the responsibility for 'health' was increasingly removed from the individual and replaced by a dependence upon medical intervention and required public health measures. Individuals were merely responsible for accessing the professional health delivery system in a timely manner. In essence the need for health care was seen as an episodic necessity -- not as a continuing individual responsibility.

Not until the latter half of this century was there a resurgence of the role and responsibility of individuals to promote and maintain their own health. Whereas therapeutic medicine had solved many of the technical problems associated with established illness, much of the illness being treated was thought to be preventable, not by drugs or medical technology, but preventable by the adoption and practice of healthy life-styles. One indication of this renewed emphasis was the establishment, in 1971, of the President's Committee on Health Education (President's Committee, 1973: 25). Subsequent to the Committee's report, the Bureau of Health Education was

Direct all communication to W. Scott Ford, Department of Sociology; Florida State University; Tallahassee, Florida. This is a revised version of a paper presented to the Society for the Study of Social Problems, Boston, 1979 and subsequently published in the Journal of Sociology and Social Welfare, Vol. 7, No. 3, May, 1980. The data were collected pursuant to a contract with the Office of Comprehensive Health Planning, Florida Department of Health and Rehabilitative Services, Tallahassee, Florida.

established within the national Center for Disease
Control. In 1974, attention was directed to public
health education as one of the ten national health
priorities cited in the National Health Planning and
Resources Development Act (U.S. Laws, 99 Stat: 2225).
Throughout the 1970s, health promotion became a topic for
national symposia; focusing on life-styles, practitioners
and scientists renewed their belief in the assumption of
individual responsibility for good health.

Florida responded to the need for more effective consumer health education by establishing a system of
regional Health Education Resource Centers (HERCs). In
1977, the state pilot program was initiated in the 18
counties of northern Florida known as the Panhandle. The
Center functions as a coordinator of area programs, an
innovator of new programs, and a clearinghouse for health
education information and materials.

THE HOUSEHOLD HEALTH SURVEY

Consumer health education is defined as the process
that informs, motivates, and helps people to adopt and
maintain healthy practices and life-styles. Perhaps the
most important questions in health education today is:
"How can we encourage/motivate people to lead healthier
lives?" And, as a correlate to this query: "What kinds
of people (in terms of attitudes, knowledge, behavior,
demographic profile) currently do or do not practice
'healthy' life-styles?" The Florida Panhandle HERC
addressed this latter question via a contract with the
authors to conduct a health education needs assessment
survey. Selected results of the survey are reported in
this article.

In the summer of 1978, a household health survey was
completed in the Florida Panhandle.[1] The household

---

[1]A multi-stage area probability sample was employed in
order to collect the household data. In order to reduce
sampling error, in the first stage of sampling, the
Panhandle counties were stratified on the basis of education, income, size of largest town, and geographic location. The largest counties (population of 40,000 or
more) were selected with certainty. Controlled probability selection was employed in order to insure geographic
dispersion of counties. In the second stage of sampling,
each county was divided into two strata -- a city directory stratum and an "area" stratum consisting of the proportion of the county not covered by the directory. The
proportion of households falling within the city directory area varied across counties, but for all counties
combined it represented approximately 75 percent. Randomly
selected areas, on the average containing approximately

interview data were readily divided into four types of items: health-related attitudes and opinions; health knowledge; health-related behaviors; and questions which taken together could provide an abbreviated health status profile.[2]

The objective of this article is to explore the impact of selected variables upon healthy life-styles. More specifically, characteristics of individuals who engage in good eating habits, exercise regularly for its own sake, do not use tobacco, and use auto safety belts are contrasted with those of their counterparts who do not routinely practice these positive health behaviors. Suggested reasons for individuals' compliant or noncompliant behaviors are given by items reflecting their demographic characteristics, predisposing attitudes, and health-related knowledge.

In preliminary analyses, a number of variables were examined individually and in combination. Several were then selected which best reflect eating habits, regular exercise, smoking behavior, and risk prevention; these variables are respectively designated "SNACK3D," SMOKE2A," "EXERCISE2," and "BELTS1." [These variables are described more fully in the note to Table 9.1] Conceptually, these four variables are considered dependent ones, reflecting respondents' compliant/noncompliant behaviors; i.e., "evidence" of a healthy/unhealthy life-style. These behaviors are chosen not only because of the number of relationships which appear between them and other predisposing attitudes, characteristics, and

---

thirty housing units, were taken to represent the nondirectory portions of counties. In all, interviews were attempted at 604 eligible households; these attempts yielded 321 fully completed interviews or a 53.5 percent response rate. Nearly half (49 percent) of the respondent-households were located in SMSA counties with populations of 50,000 or greater while 16 percent were located in "potential" SMSA counties and 35 percent were in non-urban areas (i.e., rural or small town). For a detailed discussion of the sampling procedures, see Ford and Ford (1979).

[2]Unlike the National Center for Health Statistics surveys, the HERC Survey did not obtain the same health status information for every household member. Emphasis was placed on collecting data on a large spectrum of issues -- particularly those concerning life-style variables which could only be learned from the interviewees. The respondent sought was the adult "most knowledgeable" about the health of family members: this led to a majority of female primary respondents, 78 percent (251).

knowledge, but also due to their current research relevance.[3]

EMPIRICAL FINDINGS: CORRELATES OF POSITIVE LIFE-STYLES

How prevalent are the selected behaviors in the study population? The majority (59 percent, 183) report exercising everyday/nearly everyday while 41 percent (128) do not routinely exercise; nearly half (46 percent) of the 183 'exercisers' do so for "reasons of maintaining/regaining good health." The distribution of smokers (39 precent, (121), ex-smokers (24 percent, 74), and non-smokers (37 percent, 116) is similar to that cited in a recent Surgeon General's Report.[4] Snacking is often considered a national pastime; while the majority of the sample are no exception, 40 percent (122) reportedly do not routinely snack. Included within the 60 percent (187) who do snack everyday or nearly everyday, 12 percent (37) snack only on nutritional foods, 18 percent (57) on both nutritional and 'junk' foods, and 30 percent (93) on only 'junk' foods. By self-report the majority of respondents (60 percent, 186) do not use seat belts; an additional 18 percent (57) use them only "occasionally" while 22 percent (67) use them "frequently." Frequent users are further specified into "always use" (13 percent, 40) and "often use" (9 percent, 27). Self-reported belt use is virtually identical to observed and self-

---

[3]Some recent articles examining nutrition and snacking behavior are (Abrams, 1978; Eshelman and McCloy, 1979; Fusillo and Beloian, 1977; Hansen and Wyse, 1979; Podel et al., 1978). Smoking and the correlates of this behavior have been subjected to extensive study in recent years; e.g., see (Croog and Richards, 1977; Eysenck, 1973; Foss, 1973; Jarvik et al.., 1977; Lazarsfeld, 1973; Shewchuk, 1976; Thomas, 1973; U.S. Public Health Service, 1979; and West et al., 1977). Selected articles discussing frequency, type, and/or relationship of regular exercise to health include (Gallup Onion Index, 1978; Heinzelmann and Bagley, 1970; Stalonas, Johnson, and Christ, 1978; and Young and Ismail, 1977). Use of seat belts and attempts to alter this behavior have been the subject of considerable research including (Hart Research Associates, Inc., 1978; Helsing and Comstock, 1977; Neumann et al., 1974; Opinion Research Corporation, 1978; Reisinger and Williams, 1978; Robertson et al., 1974; and Robertson, O'Neill and Wixon, 1972).
[4]While 39 percent of the sample respondents currently smoke, the Surgeon General's report estimated that 38 percent of adult males and 30 percent of adult females smoked in 1978 (U.S. Public Health Services, 1978: viii).

reported usage found in several other large scale research projects.[5]

Table 9.1 indicates the basic bivariate relationships between each of the four "behavior" variables discussed above and selected other factors. Included in this Table are all the initially hypothesized relationships. Confirmed relationships are designated by their levels of statistical significance.

TABLE 9.1
Bivariate Associations: Four Major Preventive Health Compliance Indicators by Demographic Characteristics, Predisposing Attitudes and Characteristics, and Knowledge

Independent Variables			Dependent Variables
Demographic Characteristics[a]	Predisposing Attitudes & Characteristics[b]	Knowledge[c]	Behavior[d]
***Age (-) *Educ(+) Employ Income **Nchild(+) ***Origin(+) Race	***Tensel(+) Weight	Foods ⟶ Heart2	SNACK3D
***Age(-) Educ Employ Income Nchild ***Origin(+) Race	***Clubs1(-) **Phealth(+) *Tensel(+) Threat1 **Threat2(+) *Weight(-)	Cancer7 *Cancer8(-) ⟶ ***Heart3(+)	SMOKE2A
**Age(-) **Educ(+) Employ Income *Nchild(-) Origin Race	***Exerc7(+) ***Phealth(+) ***Tensel(-) Threat2 Threat3 **Weight(-)	Heart1 ⟶	EXERC2

Table 9.1 continued....

[5]Two studies prepared for the National Highway Traffic Safety Administration report similiar findings. Based on self-report data, 25 percent of a selected sample of 2,016 adults frequently use seat belts (Hart Research Associates, Inc., 1978: 3). Based on observed usage, 14.1 percent of 68,679 adults were wearing seat belts at the time of observation (Opinion Research Corporation, 1978: 2,7).

128

Table 9.1 continued...

Age	***Phealth(+)	**Foods(+)	
***Educ(+)	***Tensel(-)	*Cancer8(+) $\longrightarrow$	BELT1
***Employ(+)	***Weight(-)	*Heart1(+)	
***Income(+)			
***Nchild(-)			
**Origin(+)			
Race			

* = .10 > p > .05, tau B/tau C
** = .05 ≥ p > .01, tau B/Tau C
*** = .01 ≥ p, tau B/tau C

aDemographic characteristics reported are age (young = 18-44; old = 45+), education (low = less than high school; moderate = high school graduate; high = post-secondary), employ (not employed outside the home; employed), income (low = less than $11,000 per year; high = $11,000 or more per year), nchild (0 = no children living in household; 1 = 1 or 2 children living in household; 2 = 3 or more children living in household), origin (1 = rural/small town community-of-origin; 2 = small city/large city community-of-origin), and race (1 = White; 2 = Black).

bPredisposing attitudes and characteristics reported are clubs1 (respondents were asked if they actively participate in any organizations, clubs, etc.), exerc7 (respondents were asked how important regular physical exercise is in keeping a person healthy), phealth (respondents were asked to evaluate the state of their own personal health compared to that of relevant others), tensel (respondents were asked how often they feel tense and nervous), threat 1, 2, and 3 (respondents were asked to identify which of five major diseases they consider to be most threatening to their own health now or in the future; threat1 = cancer; threat2 = heart attack/heart disease; threat3 = hypertension), and weight (respondents were asked if they consider themselves to be overweight and, if so, by how much).

cKnowledge items reported are foods (respondents were asked to identify the four 'basic food groups'), cancer7 and 8 (respondents were asked to name the seven warning signs of cancer; cancer7 = named nagging cough as a sign of cancer; cancer8 = total number of cancer signs correctly named), heart 1,2 and 3 (respondents were asked to cite the ways an individual could reduce his/her chances of having a heart attack/heart disease; heart 1 = named 'proper exercise'; heart 2 = named 'proper diet'; heart 3 = named not smoking).

dBehaviors include selected indicators for dietary habits (SNACKS3D = type of snacking behavior respondents engage

In reviewing Table 9.1, the strength of the demographic variables is apparent -- although many variables are not consistently related to all four beha- viors. Based on this initial analysis, what charac- teristics are associated with adoption of healthy practices? Not snacking (or nutritional snacking) is associated with each of the following attributes: older age, less education, few (or no) children, rural origin, and less tension. Non-smoking tends to be associated with older respondents, rural background, group mem- bership, a higher than average body weight (by self-report), and low levels of daily tension. Non- smokers are able to name more of the seven warning signs of cancer than are smokers. While non-smokers are less likely to feel threatened by heart attack/disease than are smokers, they are also less likely to cite 'not smoking' as a way to reduce chances of heart problems. The relationship between assessment of personal health vis-a-vis others and smoking behavior is unexpected; smo- kers tend to evaluate their own health as being better than familiar others more often than do non-smokers.

Engaging in regular exercise is associated with youth, higher levels of education, few (or no) children, average body weight, and low levels of tension. Exercisers are more likely to cite 'proper exercise' as an important way to maintain 'good health.' They also preceive their own health as better than that of relevant others. Regular seat belt use is associated with higher education, current employment, higher income, smaller family size, average body weight, and lower levels of tension. Belt users are more likely than non-belt users to assess their own health as better than others; they are also more knowledgeable about selected health matters such as knowledge of the basic four food groups and the seven warning signs of cancer.

The above highlights the selected explanatory variables, presenting an initial analysis of the major independent variables with the four health behavior dependent variables. As previously noted, the statisti- cally significant bivariate relationships are summarized in Table 9.1. Throughout the following four sections, controls are introduced to further specify the nature of these primary relationships. The results are presented without extensive comment. Implications of these

---

in; no snacks; nutritional snacks; 'junk' food); exercise (EXERC2 = whether or not respondents report exercising every day or nearly every day), smoking behavior (SMOKE2A = whether respondents currently smoke, have smoked in the past but have stopped, or have never smoked), and seat belt usage (BELTS1 = if, and how often, respondents use seat belts).

findings are reserved for the discussion section.

Snacking Behavior (SNACK3D)

SNACK3D is used as an indicator of dietary habits (see Table A1). The bivariate relationship between tension (TENSE1) and snacking is hypothesized to be a negative one (hypA); i.e., those who do not snack or snack only on nutritional foods) are less likely to report frequent high levels of tension. This relationship is confirmed; it is strongest for the older respondents, the moderately and highly educated, those with high income, respondents in families with no children living at home, individuals with an urban community-of-origin, and for whites. Not snacking is also hypothesized to be negatively associated with overweight (hypB); i.e., those who nutritionally snack (or do not snack) are less likely to be overweight. Upon analysis, this association is not statistically significant; however, when controls are introduced, the hypothesis is supported and found to be particularly strong for the following groups: older respondents, those with least education, the 'unemployed,'[6] individuals with one or two children in the home, respondents with a rural community-of-origin, and whites.

Knowing the basic four food groups (FOODS) is used as an indicator of nutritional knowledge; i.e., it is hypothesized that people who nutritionally snack (or do not snack) are more likely to identify these groups correctly (hypC). This hypothesis is not supported; in fact, the relationship is a negative one for those with a high-school education, for the employed, for the relatively high income, for those originally from rural areas, and for whites. Another knowledge item (HEART2) is hypothesized to be positively related to good eating habits (hypD). This hypothesis is also rejected; this rejection is particularly apparent for the older respondents, for those with no children living in the home, and for those with a rural community-of-origin. In summary, the preselected predisposing attitudes/characteristics are useful indicators of 'good' snacking behavior; the knowledge indicators are not.

Smoking Behavior (SMOKE2A)

SMOKE2A is used as an indicator of smoking behavior (see Table A2). The bivariate relationship between smoking and assessment of personal health compared to relevant others (PHEALTH) is hypothesized to be a positive

---

6'Unemployed' includes women who are not employed outside the home as well as the retired and other unemployed.

one (hypE). Hypothesis E is not supported even when the controls are introduced. Interestingly, there is some suggestion that non-smokers are <u>less</u> likely than smokers to assess their own health as good compared to others; this is particularly true for respondents from small households, for those with a rural community-of-origin, and for blacks. Another predisposing attitude/characteristic is tension (TENSE1); frequent high levels of tension are hypothesized to be less likely in non-smokers than in smokers (hypF). Moderate support is found for this hypothesis which is particularly strong for the young and for blacks.

Since non-smokers are practicing a 'good' health behavior, it is hypothesized that they will feel less threatened by diseases which have been directly linked to smoking; e.g., cancer and heart attack/disease. Surprisingly, the bivariate relationship between non-smoking and threat of cancer (hypG), while in the predicted negative direction, is a relatively weak one. When controls are introduced, hypG is confirmed for the old, the employed, the low income, and for those with a rural background. Further, hypG is soundly rejectd for those respondents with an urban community-of-origin; i.e., non-smokers originally from urban areas are <u>more likely</u> than their smoker counterparts to feel threatened by cancer.

Hypothesis H explores the relationship between smoking and perceived threat of heart attack/disease. As predicted, non-smokers cite fear of heart attack less often than do smokers; this is especially true for the older group, for those with less than a high school education, for the "unemployed," for the low income, for those with large families at home, for those with rural backgrounds, and for whites.

It is hypothesized that non-smokers are more knowledgeable about the signs of cancer. CANCER7 and CANCER8 are used to assess this relationship. Both hypotheses (hypI and hypJ) are weakly supported. The association between non-smoking and ability to name 'nagging cough' as a warning sign (hypI) is particularly strong within the older group and somewhat less so among blacks and among the more highly educated group. One might expect that non-smokers could name more of the seven warning signs of cancer than could smokers (hypJ). This finding is statistically significant for the older respondents, those with more years of education, the low income, those with large families still at home, individuals with rural backgrounds, and among blacks.

Non-smokers are also expected to more often cite avoidance or cessation of smoking as a means of reducing their chances of heart attack/disease (hypK). This hypothesis, if supported, would imply a direct relationship between knowledge and behavior. Rather surprisingly, hypothesis K is soundly rejected (-.000).

Additionally, this negative association remains strong even when controls are introduced. Thus, one concludes that smokers, as opposed to non-smokers, are more likely to see smoking as a direct threat to their health -- and yet persist in the habit.

Exercise (EXERC2)

EXERC2 is used as an indicator of daily/regular exercise (see Table A3). The bivariate relationship between exercise and an individual's attitude regarding the value of exercise to health (EXERC7) is hypothesized to be a positive one; i.e., those who regularly exercise are more likely to feel that exercise is important for the maintenance of good health (hypL). This association receives strong support. With the introduction of controls, the relationship is found to be especially strong across four major groups -- age, income, education, and race. Hypothesis M suggests that daily exercise is correlated with the perception of better health compared to relevant others. Again, the hypothesis is confirmed and is particularly strong for the older respondents, for those with the least education, for the low income, and for both races.

It is expected that those who exercise regularly will report lower levels of daily tension (hypN). The predicted negative relationship between tension and exercise is found to be a very strong one; it holds for all age groups and both races but is strongest for the low income and for those with a moderate amount of education.

Research suggests that the incidence of heart attacks and hypertension is reduced by regular exercise. Thus, one might anticipate that those who exercise regularly feel less threatened by these diseases. Rather unexpectedly, neither of these hypotheses (hypO and hypP) is supported. In fact, those with an urban community-of-origin are more likely to feel threatened by heart disease and engage in regular exercise. The young, the high income, and those respondents with one or two children living at home are more likely to report both engaging in regular exercise and feeling personally threatened by hypertension. Perhaps fear of these diseases (objectively justified or not) is a major contributing factor in establishing habits of regular exercise for these groups.

Finally, a knowledge item (HEART1) is studied. It is expected that people who regularly exercise are more likely to cite "proper exercise" as a means of reducing their chances of developing heart disease (hypQ). The bivariate analysis lends some weak support to this hypothesis. With controls, the relationship is found to be strong for the young, the employed, the low income, and for those with an urban community-of-origin.

In summary, the preselected predisposing attitudes/ characteristics are found to be consistent correlates of regular exercise -- with tension and perception of the importance of exercise to health being the most useful indicators of compliance in this area. Those who regularly exercise are more likely to feel threatened by heart disease and/or hypertension. By exercising, perhaps they are consciously acting to reduce this threat. The knowledge indicators are relatively weak predictors of exercise behavior.

Use of Seat Belts (BELTS1)

BELTS1 is selected as an indicator of risk prevention (see Table A4). The bivariate association between reported use of auto seat belts and one's personal health as compared to others is hypothesized to be a positive one (hypR). This hypothesis is strongly supported. It is even more strongly upheld among particular subgroups. When controls are introduced, the older respondents, those with less education, the unemployed, those from lower income families, and respondents with no children living in the household are all groups for whom the relationshp is especially significant. The association is only slightly stronger among those reared in the rural/ small town settings than for those reared in urban areas; the same small difference is found between blacks and whites.

A strong negative relationship is predicted to exist between use of seat belts and tension; i.e., those persons who report wearing seat belts will also report lower levels of daily tension (hypS). The data convincingly support this hypothesis. This finding is strongest among younger respondents, the moderately well-educated, those with higher family incomes, and those having either no children in the home or three or more. The strength and direction of this relationship is not altered by employment or community-of-origin.

It is hypothesized that people who routinely wear seat belts are also more knowledgeable in other health matters. Knowledge of the 'basic four' food groups (FOODS), the seven warning signs of cancer (CANCER8), and the relationship between exercise and reduction of heart disease are selected as measures of health knowledge. The relationship between routine seat belt use and the identification of the 'basic four' is confirmed (hypT). This relationship is particularly strong among the young, the highly educated, those without children in the household, those originally from rural areas, and among blacks. Using the second knowledge item (CANCER8), it is hypothesized that routine users of seat belts are more likely to correctly identify the seven warning signs of cancer (hypU). Whereas the relationship is in the predicted direction, it is not statistically significant. However, among white respondents and those reared in rural/small town settings, the positive relationship reaches significance.

Finally, it is suggested that persons who regularly use seat belts are more likely to designate "proper exercise" as a means of reducing their chances of developing heart attack/disease (hypV). This relationship is supported at a moderately strong level. For black respondents and for those living in households with one or two children present, the relationship is particularly strong. When family income and community-of-origin are introduced as controls, respondents with low income and those with rural backgrounds also display strong support for the hypothesis.

As is found with the three previous health behaviors (snacking, smoking, and exercise), the best indicators of seat belt usage are classified as predisposing attitudes and characteristics; two particularly important indicators are a respondent's assessment of his/her own health relative to others and the daily level of tension which the respondent reports. The relationship between general health knowledge and seat belt usage is stronger and more consistent than for the other three behaviors; yet, compared to the other predisposing factors, knowledge level is still a relatively poor correlate of positive health behavior.

DISCUSSION

What can be concluded from this analysis? What kinds of people do or do not practice 'healthy' life-styles? With regard to snacking, the stereotypes between snacking and tension and between snacking and overweight hold for whites but not for blacks. Older people who snack nutritionally (or not at all) are less likely to be overweight than older people who snack indiscriminately; however, snacking behavior in younger people does not have the same predictable effect on weight. The well-educated are more likely to report snacking that is associated with high levels of tension than are the less well-educated. Knowledge of the 'basic four' is essentially unrelated to snacking behavior. Non-nutritional snackers are more likely to identify "proper diet" as a way to reduce chances of a heart attack/disease -- exhibiting behavior in direct contradiction to their knowledge of 'appropriate' behavior.

Smoking is generally acknowledged as detrimental to health; therefore, it is disconcerting to find smokers are somewhat more likely than non-smokers to assess their own health as being better than that of relevant others. Perhaps smoking is a risk which those who perceive themselves as 'healthy' are more willing to take. That

smokers may be 'conscious risk-takers' is further suggested by the finding that smokers, more often than non-
smokers, cite 'not smoking' as a way to reduce chances of
heart disease -- another example of acting in direct
contradiction to one's 'knowledge' of what is
'appropriate' behavior. Although other research suggests
a relationship between cancer and smoking, smokers are
only slightly more likely to perceive cancer as a threat
than non-smokers. This finding may be due to a
widespread fear of cancer; however, one would expect smokers to feel this threat more acutely than non-smokers.
Smokers are appreciably more likely than non-smokers to
fear heart attacks/disease. This is particularly true of
the older group; older smokers are more likely to fear
heart disease than their age peers who do not smoke.

Regular exercise is associated in most people's minds
with general physical fitness. People who exercise regularly are more likely to value their own health and to
rate their own health as being better than others.
Discovering this association is not surprising; however,
the specifications of the primary relationship is of
particular interest; older persons who exercise assess
their health as being better than others much more often
than do older non-exercisers. Similar relationships are
found for the less well-educated as compared to the well-
educated and for the low income relative to the high
income. The older, the low income, and the less well-
educated are often of special concern to health educators. These groups are often cited for non-compliance.
It appears that, when (and if) members of these groups
are compliant, they become committed to their behavior.
Commitment to exercise is also evident in the specifica-
tion of the bivariate relationship between exercise and
attitude toward exercise (EXERC7); people who exercise
see exercise as instrumental in keeping them healthy -- a
relationship which is as strong for the low income as for
the high income, as strong for blacks as for whites,
as strong for the young as for the older group, and as
strong for the less well-educated as for the well-
educated. Thus, regular exercise is perceived as an
instrumental behavior; if one exercises, one will be
healthier. Release of tension is often seen as a benefit
of regular exercise; the data confirm a negative relationship between tension and exercise. This is particularly true for the low income and holds across age,
education, and racial groups.

Similiar to daily exercise, routine use of auto
safety belts requires a continuing and active commitment
to the maintenance of good health -- in this instance, by
reducing injury from accidents. Unlike smokers ("the
conscious risk-takers"), seat belt users are more consistently found to hold health-related attitudes which
confirm original expectations. Additionally, among belt

wearers, the relationship between using belts and health-related knowledge items is consistently in the direction expected. Particularly striking is the strong association between seat belt use and a positive assessment of one's own health relative to others. Perhaps 'buckling up' assures belt wearers that their positive assessment is a realistic one, enhancing the likelihood of maintaining their good health. Correspondingly, seat belt users are less likely than non-users to report frequent high levels of daily tension.

This analysis has identified some of the characteristics of those who live (or do not live) the "good" life. Knowledge of these characteristics should bring us somewhat closer to answering the question: "How can we encourage/motivate people to lead healthier lives?" Initially it was hoped that the data would be used to construct a dichotomy of those who practice good health behaviors and those who do not. Ideally, attributes of these groups would be identified that would be consistently related to all four types of behavior. Although these expectations were not fully realized, the data suggest a number of interesting relationships worthy of further consideration.

Looking only at those who currently engage in good health practices, consistency among these behaviors is examined. Discouragingly, it is concluded that very few people consistently practice healthy life-styles; i.e., persons who regularly engage in all four health-related behaviors comprise less than 10 percent of the respondents. However, using the tau B and tau C tests of association, consistent associations are found among several of the health behaviors. For example, if a non-snacker does not smoke, there is a strong likelihood that she/he will wear seat belts (.04). Similarly, if a non-smoker exercises regularly, she/he will routinely wear a seat belt (.04); if a non-smoker wears a seat belt, she/he will probably not snack (.04). For ex-smokers, knowing that she/he wears a seat belt will decrease the likelihood that indiscriminate snacking takes place (.01). For exercisers, consistent associations between behaviors also exist but they are less strong. If a regular exerciser does not smoke, she/he probably wears seat belts (.07); if a regular exerciser wears seat belts, she/he is less likely to snack (.10). Finally, looking only at seat belt users, if one does not smoke, one is unlikely to snack with regularity (.07).

Throughout the analysis, the one independent variable that is clearly and consistently related to all four health behaviors is that of self-reported levels of daily tension. Low levels of tension are positively related to non-snacking, non-smoking, regular exercise and the use of auto seat belts. Of course, the causal direction of these relationships is exceedingly difficult to tease out;

the current analysis assumes tension to be a predisposing condition -- an independent variable.

Conclusions derived from the analysis reported here must be regarded as exploratory. Most research in the health area focuses upon correlates of one health-related problem or behavior (one dependent variable). Whereas attempts to identify consistent adoption across several health behaviors is difficult, nevertheless further efforts in this direction are warranted. The identification of similarities and dissimilarities within and between behavior consistent groups is central to extending knowledge of 'who practices the good life?'

REFERENCES

Abrams, I.J.
    1978   "Determining Consumer Demand and Marketing Opportunities for Nutritional Products." Food Technology: 79-85.
Becker, Marshall H. and Lois A. Maiman
    1975   "Sociobehavioral Determinants of Compliance with Health and Medical Care Recommendations." Medical Care 13: 10-24.
Berkanovic, Emil
    1976   "Behavioral Science and Prevention." Preventive Medicine 5: 92-105.
Croog, Sydney H. and Nancy P. Richards
    1977   "Health Beliefs and Smoking Patterns in Heart Patients and Their Wives: A Longitudinal Study." American Journal of Public Health 67: 921-930.
Eshelman, Ruth E. and Katherine McCloy
    1979   "The Changing Face of Community Nutrition." Family and Community Health" The Journal of Health Promotion and Maintenance 1: 1-6.
Eysenck, H. J.
    1973   "Personality and the Maintenance of the Smoking Habit." Pp. 113-146 in William L. Dunn, Jr. (ed.), Smoking Behavior: Motives and Incentives. Washington, D.C.: V. H. Winston and Sons.
Ford, W. Scott and Ann S. Ford
    1979   Health Education Assessment Survey: The Florida Panhandle. Atlanta, Georgia: Bureau of Health Education, U.S. Department of Health, Education and Welfare.
Foss, Robert
    1973   "Personality, Social Influence and Cigarette Smoking." Journal of Health and Social Behavior 14: 279-286.
Fuchs, Victor R.
    1974   Who Shall Live? New York: Basic Books.

Fusillo, Alice E. and Arletta M. Beloian
    1977   "Consumer Nutrition Knowledge and Self
            Reported Food Shopping Behavior." American
            Journal of Public Health 67: 846-850.
Gallup Opinion Index
    1978   "Nearly Half of Americans Now Exercising
            Daily; 24 Percent Are Joggers." Gallup
            Opinion Index: Report number 151.
Haggerty, Robert J.
    1977   "Changing Lifestyles to Improve Health."
            Preventive Medicine 6: 276-289.
Hansen, R. Gaurth and Bonita W. Wyse
    1979   "Planning for the Inevitable: Snack Foods in
            the Diet." Family and Community Health: The
            Journal of Health Promotion and Maintenance
            1: 31-39.
Hart Research Associates, Inc.
    1978   Public Attitudes Toward Passive Restraint
            Systems: Summary Report. Washington, D.C.:
            National Highway Traffic Safety
            Administration, U.S. Department of
            Transportation.
Heinzelman, Fred and Richard W. Bagley
    1970   "Response to Physical Activity Programs and
            Their Effects on Health Behavior." Public
            Health Reports 85: 905-911.
Helsing, Knud J. and George W. Comstock
    1977   "What Kinds of People Do Not Use Seat Belts."
            American Journal of Public Health 67:
            1043-1050.
Jarvik, Murray E., Joseph W. Cullen, Ellen R. Gritz,
        Thomas M. Vogt and Louis Jolyon West (eds.)
    1977   Research on Smoking Behavior. NIDA Research
            Monograph 17. Washington, D.C.: U.S.
            Government Printing Office.
Lazarsfeld, P. F.
    1973   "The Social Sciences and The Smoking
            Problem." Pp. 283-286 in William L. Dunn,
            Jr. (ed.), Smoking Behavior: Motives and
            Incentives. Washington, D.C.: V.H. Winstong
            and Sons.
Neumann, Charlotte G., Alfred K. Neumann, Margaret E.
        Cockrell and Sheila Banani
    1974   "Factors Associated With Child Use of
            Automobile Restraining Devices." American
            Journal of Diseases of Children 128: 469-474.
Opinion Research Corporation
    1978   Safety Belt Usage: Survey of Cars in the
            Traffic Population (November 1977-June 1978).
            Washington, D.C.: National Highway Traffic
            Safety Administration, U.S. Department of
            Transportation.

Podell, Richard N., Kathryn Keller, Michael N. Mulvihill, Gary Berger and Donald Kent
    1978   "Evaluation of the Effectiveness of a High School Course in Cardiovascular Nutrition." American Journal of Public Health 68: 573-576.
President's Committee on Health Education
    1973   Report. Washington, D.C.: U.S. Government Printing Office.
Reisinger, Keith S. and Allan F. Williams
    1978   "Evaluation of Programs Designed to Increase Protection of Infants in Cars." Pediatrics 62: 280-287.
Robertson, Leon S., Albert B. Kelley, Brian O'Neill, Charles W. Wixom, Richard S. Eiswirth and William Haddon
    1974   "A Controlled Study of the Effect of Television Messages on Safety Belt Use." American Journal of Public Health 64: 1071-1080.
Robertson, Leon S., Brian O'Neill and Charles W. Wixom
    1972   "Factors Associated with Observed Safety Belt Use." Journal of Health and Social Behavior 13: 18-24.
Schewchuk, L. A.
    1976   "Smoking Cessation Programs of the American Health Foundation." Preventive Medicine 5: 454-474.
Somers, Anne R. (ed.)
    1976   Promoting Health. Germantown, Maryland: Aspen Systems Corporation.
Stalonas, Peter M., William G. Johnson and Maryann Christ
    1978   "Behavior Modification for Obesity: The Evaluation of Exercise, Contingency Management, and Program Adherence." Journal of Consulting and Clinical Psychology 46: 463-469.
Thomas, C. B.
    1973   "The Relationship of Smoking and Habits of Nervous Tension." Pp. 157-170 in William L. Dunn, Jr. (ed.), Smoking Behavior: Motives and Incentives. Washington, D.C.: V.H. Winston and Sons.
U.S. Laws, Statutes
    1974   "National Health Planning and Resources Development Act of 1974." Public Law 93-641. 88 STAT. 2225.
U.S. Public Health Service
    1979   Smoking and Health: A Report of the Surgeon General. Washington, D.C.: U.S. Government Printing Office.

140

West, Dee W., Saxon Graham, Mya Swanson and Gregg
          Wilkinson
    1977   "Five Year Follow-Up of a Smoking Withdrawal
            Clinic Population." American Journal of
            Public Health 67: 536-544.
Young, R. John and A. H. Ismail
    1977   "Comparison of Selected Physiological and
            Personality Variables in Regular and
            Nonregular Adult Male Exercisers." The
            Research Quarterly 48: 617-622.

Table A1. Snacking Behavior Controlling For Major Demographic Characteristics

Snacking Behavior (SNACK3D)

Hypothesis A: Nutritional snacking (or not snacking) is negatively associated with tension.

I. Level of Daily Tension (TENSE1)

Bivariate: -.001, strong support of hypothesis A

Hypothesis A supported:

By Age: Young*, Old***
By Education: H.S.***, > H.S.***
By Employment: Employed**, "unemployed"**
By Income: Low*, High**
By NChild: No children living in home**
            3+ children living in home*
By Origin: Rural/Small Town*, Urban***
Ry Race: White***

Hypothesis A rejected:

No significant relationships

Hypothesis B: Nutritional snacking (or not snacking) is negatively associated with overweight.

II. Weight (WEIGHT)

Bivariate: -N.S., direction suggests weak support of hypothesis B

Hypothesis B supported:

By Age: Old**
By Education: < H.S.*
By Employment: "unemployed"*
By NChild: 1 or 2 children living in home*
By Origin: Rural/Small Town*
By Race: White**

Hypothesis B rejected:

No significant relationships

Hypothesis C: People who regularly snack on nutritional foods (or do not snack) are more likely
               to know the four major food groups.

III. Basic Four Food Groups (FOODS)

Bivariate: -N.S., direction suggests weak rejection of hypothesis C

Hypothesis C supported:

No significant relationships

Hypothesis C rejected:

By Education: H.S.**
By Employment: Employed*
By Income: High**
By Origin: Rural/Small Town*
By Race: White***

Hypothesis D: People who regularly snack on nutritional foods (or do not snack) are more likely
               to identify proper diet as a way to reduce their chances of heart attack/diseases.

IV. Heart Problem & Diet (HEART2)

Bivariate: -N.S., direction suggests weak rejection of hypothesis D

Hypothesis D supported:

No significant relationships

Hypothesis D rejected:

By Age: Old**
By NChild: No children living in home**
By Origin: Rural/Small Town

```
 *    .10 ≩ p > .05, tau B/tau C
 **   .05 ≩ p > .01, tau B/tau C
 ***  .01 ≩ p, tau B/tau C
```

Table A2.   Smoking Behavior Controlling for Major Demographic Characteristics

Smoking Behavior (SMOKE2A)

Hypothesis E: Non-smokers are more likely to assess their own personal health as being better than relevant others.

I.   Personal Health Compared to Others
     (PHEALTH)   Bivariate: -N.S., direction suggests weak rejection of hypothesis E

     Hypothesis E supported: No significant relationships

     Hypothesis E rejected: By NChild: No children living in home*
                                           By Origin: Rural/Small Town*
                                           By Race: Black**

Hypothesis F: Non-smokers are less likely to report high levels of tension.

II. Level of Daily Tension (TENSE1)   Bivariate: -.08, moderate support of hypothesis F

     Hypothesis F supported: By Age: Young*
                                           By Race: Black**

     Hypothesis F rejected: No significant relationships

Hypothesis G: Non-smokers are less likely to perceive cancer as a personal threat now or in the future.

III. Cancer as Personal Threat (THREAT1)   Bivariate: -N.S., direction suggests weak support of hypothesis G

     Hypothesis G supported: By Age: Old*
                                           By Employment: Employed***
                                           By Income: Low**
                                           By Origin: Rural/Small Town***

     Hypothesis G rejected: By Origin: Urban***

Hypothesis H: Non-smokers are less likely to perceive heart attack/disease as a personal threat now or in the future.

IV. Heart Attack/Disease as a Personal
     Threat (THREAT2)   Bivariate: -.04, strong support of hypothesis H

     Hypothesis H supported: By Age: Old***
                                           By Education: < H.S.**
                                           By Employment: "Unemployed"*
                                           By Income: Low***
                                           By NChild: 3+ children living in home*
                                           By Origin: Rural/Small Town**
                                           By Race: White*

     Hypothesis H rejected: No significant relationships

Hypothesis I: Non-smokers are more likely to cite a 'nagging cough' as one of the seven signs of cancer.

V.   'Nagging Cough' as Warning Sign of
     Cancer (CANCER7)   Bivariate: +N.S., direction suggests weak support of hypothesis I

     Hypothesis I supported: By Age: Old**
                                           By Education: > H.S.*
                                           By Race: Black*

     Hypothesis I rejected: No significant relationships

Hypothesis J: Non-smokers are more likely to correctly name more of the seven warning signs of cancer.

VI. Seven Warning Signs of Cancer
     (CANCER8)   Bivariate: +.08, moderate support of hypothesis J

     Hypothesis J supported: By Age: Old**
                                           By Education: > H.S.**
                                           By Income: Low*
                                           By NChild: 3+ children living in home*
                                           By Origin: Rural/Small town***
                                           By Race: Black**

     Hypothesis J rejected: No significant relationships

Hypothesis K. Non-smokers are more likely to cite 'not smoking' as a way to reduce chances of heart attack/disease.

VII. Heart Problems and Smoking
     (HEART3)   Bivariate: -.000, strong rejection of hypothesis K

     Hypothesis K supported: No significant relationships

     Hypothesis K rejected: By Age: Young***, Old**
                                           By Education: > H.S.**, H.S.***
                                           By Employment: Employed***, "Unemployed"***
                                           By Income: Low**, High***
                                           By NChild: No children living in home***, 1 or 2 children
                                                       living in home***, 3+ children living in home**
                                           By Origin: Rural/Small Town***, Urban**
                                           By Race: White***, Black***

---

    * = .10 ≥ p > .05, tau B/tau C
   ** = .05 ≥ p > .01, tau B/tau C
  *** = .01 ≥ p, tau B/tau C

Table A3. Exercise Controlling for Major Demographic Characteristics

Exercise (EXERC2)

Hypothesis L: People who exercise regularly are more likely to feel that exercise is important for maintaining good health.

I. Attitude toward Exercise (EXERC7)   Bivariate: +.002, strong support of hypothesis L

Hypothesis L supported: By Age: Young***, Old***
                                     By Education: < H.S.***, H.S.**, > H.S.**
                                     By Income: Low***, High**
                                     By Race: White***, Black**

Hypothesis L rejected: No significant relationships

Hypothesis M: People who exercise regularly are more likely to assess their own personal health as being better than relevant others.

II. Personal Health Compared to
Others (PHEALTH)   Bivariate: +.005, strong support of hypothesis M

Hypothesis M supported: By Age: Old**
                                     By Education: < H.S.***
                                     By Income: Low*
                                     By Race: White**, Black**

Hypothesis M rejected: No significant relationships

Hypothesis N: People who exercise regularly are less likely to report high levels of tension.

III. Level of Daily Tension (TENSE1) Bivariate: -.001, strong support of hypothesis N

Hypothesis N supported: By Age: Young***, Old**
                                     By Education: < H.S.**, H.S.***
                                     By Income: Low***
                                     By Race: White***, Black**

Hypothesis N rejected: No significant relationships

Hypothesis O: People who exercise regularly are less likely to perceive heart attack/disease as a personal threat now or in the future.

IV. Heart Attack/Disease as a
Personal Threat (THREAT2)   Bivariate: + N.S.,direction suggests weak rejection of hypothesis O

Hypothesis O supported: No significant relationships

Hypothesis O rejected: By Origin: Urban**

Hypothesis P: People who exercise regularly are less likely to perceive hypertension as a personal threat now or in the future.

V. Hypertension as a Personal
Threat (THREAT3)   Bivariate: + N.S., direction suggests weak rejection of hypothesis P

Hypothesis P supported: No significant relationships

Hypothesis P rejected: By Age: Young**
                                     By Income: High***
                                     By NChild: 1 or 2 children living in home**

Hypothesis Q: People who exercise regularly are more likely to cite 'proper exercise' as a way to reduce their chances of heart attack/disease.

VI. Heart Problem & Exercise
(HEART1)   Bivariate: + N.S., direction suggests weak support of hypothesis Q

Hypothesis Q supported: By Age: Young**
                                     By Employment: Employed*
                                     By Income: Low*
                                     By Origin: Urban***

Hypothesis Q rejected: No significant relationships

  * .10 $\geq$ p > .05, tau B/tau C
 ** .05 $\geq$ p > .01, tau B/tau C
*** .01 $\geq$ p, tau B/tau C

Table A4. Seat Belt Use Controlling for Major Demographic Characteristics

Seat Belt Use (BELTS1)

Hypothesis R: People who routinely use seat belts are more likely to assess their own health
as being better than relevant others.

I. Personal Health Compared
    to Others (PHEALTH)   Bivariate: +.01, strong support of hypothesis R

    Hypothesis R supported: By Age: Old***
                                       By Education: < H.S.***
                                       By Employment: "Unemployed"***
                                       By Income: Low**
                                       By NChild: No children living in home***, 1 or 2 children
                                                  living in home*

    Hypothesis R rejected: No significant relationships

Hypothesis S: People who routinely use seat belts are less likely to report high levels of tension.

II. Level of Daily Tension (TENSE1)   Bivariate: -.01, strong support of hypothesis S

    Hypothesis S supported: By Age: Young***
                                       By Education: < H.S.*, H.S.**
                                       By Employment: Employed**, "Unemployed"**
                                       By Income: High***
                                       By NChild: No children living in home**, 3+ children living
                                                  in home***
                                       By Origin: Rural/Small Town**, Urban**

    Hypothesis S rejected: No significant relationships

Hypothesis T: People who routinely use seat belts are more likely to know the four major food groups.

III. Basic Four Food Groups (FOODS)   Bivariate: +.02, strong support of hypothesis T

    Hypothesis T supported: By Age: Young**
                                       By Education: < H.S.***
                                       By Employment: "Unemployed"*
                                       By Income: Low*
                                       By NChild: No children living in home**
                                       By Origin: Rural/Small Town**
                                       By Race: White*, Black**

    Hypothesis T rejected: No significant relationships

Hypothesis U: People who routinely use seat belts are more likely to correctly name more of
the seven warning signs of cancer.

IV. Seven Warning Signs of Cancer
    (CANCER8)   Bivariate: +.10, direction suggests weak support of hypothesis U

    Hypothesis U supported: By Origin: Rural/Small Town*
                                       By Race: White**

    Hypothesis U rejected: No significant relationships

Hypothesis V: People who routinely use seat belts are more likely to cite 'proper exercise'
as a way to reduce their chances of heart attack/disease.

V. Heart Problems & Exercise
    (HEART1   Bivariate: +.07, moderate support of hypothesis V

    Hypothesis V supported: By Income: Low*
                                       By NChild: 1 or 2 children living in home***
                                       By Origin: Rural*
                                       By Race: Black***

    Hypothesis V rejected: No significant relationships

*   .10 ≥ p > .05, tau B/tau C
**   .05 ≥ p > .01, tau B/tau C
*** .01 ≥ p, tau B/tau C

10
The Impact of Consumerism on Health Care Change: Alternatives for the Future?

Allen W. Imershein   Florida State University
Eugenia T. Miller   University of California

The quest for consumer participation in the management of health care delivery may have experienced its first signs of success, but the implications of that success are as yet unclear. The establishment of consumer majorities on health systems agency (HSA) boards was seen as an important milestone in the development of the consumer movement in America over the last ten years. The initial wave of optimism over the Great Society programs that in part gave birth to the consumer movement has long since vanished, but some of the organizational results of those attempts at innovation have become routinely established, as the requirements for consumer participation specified in wave after wave of health related amendments clearly indicates. But what are the results of this participation, and what can we reasonably expect in the future?

Many of the initial problems of consumer involvement remain with us, especially where lay consumers and expert professional serve together in the same organizational setting, as is typically the case. Providers dominate decision-making despite the presence of consumer majorities on decision-making bodies. Critics have questioned the naivete which suggested that simple consumer involvement would provide some measure of public accountability. Evidence thus far clearly demonstrates that such is not the case (Navarro, 1973; Metsch and Veney, 1976). Critics have also suggested, however, that these problems are not insurmountable and that, with some revisions in the program for consumer participation, the power and control may shift from the provider to the consumer realm, as consumer ideology has all along claimed it should. The discussion to follow will argue that even if the problems of participation are surmounted· and if consumers do gain greater control of relevant boards and councils, the net effect will not be to shift control of health care organization from providers to consumers. Rather, given the present organizational arrangements and opportunities, the effect would be to shift the control of health care delivery from one group of providers to another.

THE UNCERTAIN GROWTH OF CONSUMERISM IN HEALTH CARE

The growth of consumerism in American society has sometimes been hailed as a new social movement (Reeder, 1972). Sparked by the emergence of consumer involvement in OEO-sponsored neighborhood health centers, the development of the movement in health care has been fostered by the beginning redefinition of roles -- from doctor-patient to provider-consumer, by a shift in concern from curative and crisis care to preventive care, by the change from solo practice to bureaucratic models for delivery which more readily provide organizational avenues for consumer involvement, and, of course, by the overall legislative support granted to consumer participation (Reeder, 1972, Milio, 1974). But the organizational success thus far has been mixed at best (Stoller, 1974; Metsch and Veney, 1976; Douglass, 1975). Consumers may have moved into the decision-making realm, but their impact within this realm has been limited. The factors which have been cited to explain this limited impact can be grouped into three main categories.

First, consumers have been seen as largely unprepared for their new roles. Despite the fact that they are now labeled "consumers" rather than "patients," they tend to regard the providers as the only ones having the necessary expertise to make important decisions. Thus, whatever viewpoint they may bring to the setting, that perspective becomes coopted in favor of that of the providers. Moreover, consumers are often inexperienced in speaking out in committee contexts and therefore less able to articulate a position which might be controversial (Stoller, 1974). Finally, the extent to which consumers have a clearly legitimated role to take the control which their majority status would make possible is at best unclear (Maxmen, 1976).

Second, providers have a clearly vested interest in maintaining control in all organizational settings which affect their everyday work practices. Participation on committees is viewed as one part of already well-defined professional roles in contrast to the largely voluntary status of consumers. Providers may be willing to allow consumer input over relatively minor issues, but will structure committee action in such a way as to defer or define in their own terms issues of critical concern (Milio, 1974; Stoller, 1975; cf. Bachrach and Baratz, 1970; Warren et al, 1974).

Third, a number of "system" characteristics would tend not to encourage the development of consumer strength. The legislative mandate, though clearly placing consumers in a majority status, failed to define clear role activities for that participation (Metsch and

Veney, 1976). Existing resources which might be used in decision-making are much more available to providers than consumers. Few situations outside the immediate context provide occasions in which consumers might coalesce into an organized group or articulate proposals and arguments, i.e., the organizational superiority of providers is clearly evident.

Finally, the placement of consumers on advisory and management boards serves to legitimate the continued decision-making of these groups without necessarily changing the character of the decisions or important decision-makers. Thus, weak consumer participation contributes to the maintenance of the "system" without fundamentally changing it (Navarro, 1973; 1976). Consumer participation, as Metsch and Veney (1976) suggest, is indeed good politics.

Critical commentaries on the problems of consumer participation have also proposed a number of solutions to aid that process (Young, 1975; Stoller, 1974; Milio, 1974; Friedson, 1970). The development of organizational and leadership experiences for consumers is seen to be crucial. Resources need to be made more available. Tasks need to be better defined. Further legislation needs to set forth clear role responsibilities. Providers need to be persuaded of both the importance and usefulness of more than token consumer participation. The legitimation of consumer decision-making as an inherent right needs to be solidly established. And con-sumers need to be better educated, better organized and more certain of their own investment in these new orga-nizational roles (Illich, 1976).

STRUCTURAL BARRIERS TO CHANGE

Despite the optimism conveyed by those supporters of consumer based programs, the variety of proposed resolu-tions to problems of consumer participation must finally be seen as naive and largely superficial. To be sure, the development of resources, specified roles, leadership experience, provider indulgence, and the like, will make for a stronger consumer voice on decision-making boards. But what will be the position spoken for in this newly-gained realm? Arguments rejecting provider dominance assume that consumers have a well-defined and agreed upon position from which to speak. Evidence suggests the contrary. Consumers disagree widely over who should engage in decision-making activities, how much government should be involved in the financing of health care, and whether there is even a problem to be dealt with (Strasmann, 1975). Moreover, this disagreement over major issues may reflect a more fundamental factor explaining the lack of consumer consensus: the lack of a stuctural base which could unify consumer interests and organize their efforts.

Alford (1975) has argued that the current health care controversy can be understood as reflecting political and organizational maneuvering among long-standing structural interests, which represent professional, legislative, and cultural institutional arangements. The professional monopoly of private physicians, their organizations, and the laws and customs surrounding their activities constitute the major structural interest which has dominated American health care for the last fifty years. The changing technology and division of labor in health care in recent years created basic conflicts with these dominant practices and has yielded a second structural interest based on hospitals, public health and health planning organizations, and the corporate sector supporting much of these activities. Indicative of this new structual interest has been the emergence of a bureaucratic reform movement calling for an end to fragmented care, for greater coordination and integration of services, and for more continuity and comprehensiveness in the provision of care, all of which would be enhanced by better management and regulation, i.e., the development of bureaucratic medicine (Mechanic, 1976). Alford recognizes a third structural interest, that of the consumer population, but he characterizes it as repressed, for "no social institutions or political mechanisms in the society insure that these interests are served" (1975:15). Consumers may have power in numbers, but without an institutional base which would serve to recognize those numbers, they are unlikely to affect the present system.

Warren's (1974) data on community decision organizations provides some additional confirmation for Alford's perspective. These organizations by and large focused on delivery of services to what was seen as a poverty population in need of aid. Even without the provision of explicit rules, the dominant "institutionalized thought structure," as Warren calls it (similar to Alford's structural interests), provided for consistent action across both differing organizations and differing cities. When a challenge was mounted against this dominant structure, and power was shifted to a new group, the activities carried out in the newly controlled organizational settings differed little from those of the previous group, despite an outpouring of ideological rhetoric. In other words, lacking a concrete strategy for action, challenging groups tended to redefine the problem in terms of existing means for "problem-solving." In similar fashion, the consumer movement in health care may be little more than good rhetoric for those out of power and good politics for those who are in.

POSSIBLE ALTERNATIVES

The explanation we have provided above may prove tempting to both critical and cynical observers of the American political and health care scenes. Though it is undoubtedly more accurate than the largely optimistic viewpoints noted earlier, it may at the same time deny an important aspect of the consumer movement in health care. Although we have argued that health care consumerism consists mainly of ideology and lacks a structural base, the movement is not totally without substance. But the substantive nature of the arguments proposed by consumer advocates may lead along different paths than those advocates presume. These arguments divide the advocates into two broad and not necessarily overlapping groups. That the two groups may have ultimately conflicting goals (cf. Starr, 1976) makes it essential that further research and discussion take note of the distinguishing characteristics.

The first group is the most vocal and pushes the most heavily for fundamental change (see for example, Heal Yourself or The American Health Empire). Their arguments focus upon the continuing health care crisis, in particular, the maldistribution of resources -- hospitals, physicians and the like, the fragmentation of the health care system, the improper locus of control, the search for profits, the conflict of interest positions of providers, the discrimination against the poor and racial minorities. Not all critiques name all these elements, by any means, but there is considerable overlap. As an alternative to the present system, most of the above elements need to be reversed. The health care system needs to be accesssible and responsive to consumers, and consumers need to be in decision-making positions to insure that possibility. The system needs to be organized to provide coordinated care that is comprehensive in nature; preventive as well as crisis care; providers need to be removed from conflict of interest positions, and the profit-making motive needs to be eliminated. How is all this to be accomplished? Presumably the development of a consumer-oriented, consumer controlled system would do just that. But is this claim anything more than ideological rhetoric with no possibility of occurrence as Alford and others suggest?

If it is more than rhetoric, then the fulfillment of these claims will likely not take the course entirely consistent with the proposed arguments. It is striking that proposals for change emerging from the consumer movement are very similar to those from the bureaucratic reform movement noted earlier: a critique of the fragmented and maldistributed system; a call for greater integration, coordination, comprehensiveness, and continuity of care, i.e., calls for better regulation and management of the current system. Given the nature of the proposed changes and the size and complexity of the current system, it is unlikely that anyone other than a managerial group, i.e., the "corporate bureaucrats," would take charge of such changes. Thus in both rhetoric and effect, this aspect of the consumer movement can be seen as no more than an extension of the already ongoing bureaucratic reform movement (Navarro, 1973, 1976). The process of change might supply more rules for consumers than ever before, but the substance would result in a shift of power not to the consumers, but instead from one group of providers, the professional monopolists, to another, the corporate bureaucrats. In that sense, the consumer movement is good politics indeed.

The second group in the consumer movement may seem less vocal than the first. They comprise the varied range of participants in what might be called the self-care movement (see especially Levin et al, 1976). Their major thrust is not toward changing the current health care system, but toward minimizing the need for it. Whatever the organizational strengths or weaknesses of the current system, it is seen by this group as oriented toward sick care rather than health. In contrast to the professionally based expertise requisite for the sick care system, the wellness orientation of the self care movement emphasizes lay responsibility, both individual and group (Carlson, 1975). Such an orientation is manifest in the feminist health center development, the emergence of some of the free clinics, and growth of nutritional awareness and interest in "health foods," and the calls for reliance on the natural healing powers of the body and the pomotion of natural ways of living and interacting with one's environment (see e.g., Samuels and Bennett, 1973; The Boston Women's Health Collective, 1972; see also Levin et al, 1976,: 94-114 for annotated bibliography).

The self-care movement, if it is yet in fact a movement (Levin et al, 1976: 31ff), must be distinguished from a broader ideology which has recently gained considerable currency. On the one hand this ideology, exemplified by the arguments of Ivan Illich (1976), rejects the medical care system in toto as doing more to cause than to cure sickness, a view congruent with an earlier "therapeutic nihilism" (cf. Starr, 1976). On the other and complimentary hand, it emphasizes the importance of individual reliance and self-help groups, here construed more broadly than an application solely to health. This ideology has been roundly criticized for its rejection of considerable successes in the medical care system, its conflicting goals for better health, and its uninformed attitude toward larger structural issues affecting health (Fox, 1977; Starr, 1976; Sidel and Sidel, 1976; among many).

Whatever strength exists in the self-care movement does not lie in the strident ideology noted above, however, but in a set of day-to-day practices which emphasize the growth and utilization of lay medical knowledge rather than the rejection of professional expertise and the centrality of individual responsibility and life-style choices rather than the irrelevance of the medical care system. The extent to which professional knowledge and the medical care system are de-emphasized results from an awareness that a reliance on these does not necessarily promote health but primarily cures sickness. Such a stance is consistent with long-standing public health and a recent more general perception of the relative lack of impact of the medical care system on health levels of the population in comparision with broader social and environmental changes (see e.g., Lalonde, 1974; Fuchs, 1974; Levin et al, 1976; Task Force on Preventive Medicine, 1976; Daedalus, Winter, 1977, passim).

The efforts of this group parallel a growing shift from curative medicine to preventive medicine with atten- dant emphasis on health education and health promotion at an early age (cf. Carlson, 1975). While curative medi- cine relegates the consumer to the passive role of patient, preventive medicine promotes an active orien- tation toward personal health maintenance (Morse, 1979). There is ample evidence that such a shift is occurring. For example, efforts to curtail smoking, the rapidly growing interest in exercise, breast self-examinations, among others, point to an increased acceptance of per- sonal responsibility for maintaining one's own health. This movement is further highlighted in the diffusion of medical technology to lay consumers as evidenced in the marketing of self-administered pregnancy test kits and personal blood pressure cuffs that allow for self- monitoring. Relatedly, current efforts to minimize environmental health hazards, both within the work environment as well as in the broader environment, speak to a burgeoning consumer concern with averting future health hazards. Recent organized protests against con- tinued operation and new building of nuclear power plants have dramatized such active concerns. We suggest that this new kind of consumer activism, both in the promotion of self-care and in the prevention of environmental health hazards, is gaining broad socio-cultural support. By and large, these efforts may mark the beginning of an undermining of what Starr (1978: 177) has called the "cultural authority of medicine."

Given this more personalized orientation, it is surprising that its advocates are not seen in the forefront of those working for change in the current medical care system. However, this latter branch of the consumer movement may have more long-range impact than the former. For unlike the former, this group is based on a set of everyday practices closely related to changing attitudes about health maintenance around which a strong and coherent movement could arise. It is the new practices which may prove essential in any significant social change (cf. Imershein, 1977a, 1977b). Its declaration of relative independence from the current system, while not totally rejecting it, may serve to provide greater possibilities for the development of power than one which attempts to modify the system. The success of such a movement would not be registered by organizational changes which could be co-opted by more powerful groups, as would be the case with the organizational reform group noted earlier. Its co-optation by the current system, if possible, might register its success: the redistribution of specialized medical knowledge and responsibility for health. Thus the impact could be more broadly cultural and more clearly long-range. It may resemble the previous turn of the century medical revolution which took more than thirty years to accomplish, while at the same time reversing the flow of knowledge accomplished by that revolution. In this respect it may be seen as the development of a new approach to health care which may in the end impact the existing organization of health care delivery by gradually diffusing its power base and thus weakening the existing professional monopoly.

REFERENCES

Alford, Robert R.
   1975   Health Care Politics: Ideological and Interest Group Barriers to Reform. Chicago: University of Chicago Press.

Bachrach, P. and M. Baratz
   1970   Power and Poverty. New York: Oxford University Press.

Bodenheimer, T., S. Cummings, and F. Harding (eds.)
   1972   Billions for Bandaids. San Francisco: Medical Committee for Human Rights.

The Boston Women's Health Collective
   1971   Our Bodies, Ourselves. New York: Simon & Schuster.

Carlson, Rick J.
   1975   The End of Medicine. New York: John Wiley & Sons.

Citizens Board of Inquiry into Health Services for Americans
   1972   Heal Yourself. Washington: The American Public Health Association.

Daedalus
   1977   "Doing Better and Feeling Worse: Health in the U.S." Special Issue. Daedalus 106, No. 1.

Douglass, Chester W.
    1975   "Consumer Influence in Health Planning in the
            Urban Ghetto." Inquiry 12 (June): 157-163.
Ehrenreich, Barbara and John Ehrenreich
    1970   The American Health Empire. New York: Random
            House
Fox, Renee C.
    1977   "The Medicalization and Demedicalization of
            American Society." Daedalus 106 (Winter):
            9-22.
Friedson, Eliot
    1970   Profession of Medicine: A Study of the
            Sociology of Applied Knowledge. New York:
            Dodd, Mead & Co.
Fuchs, Victor
    1974   Who Shall Live? New York: Basic Books
Illich, Ivan
    1976   Medical Nemesis: The Expropriation of Health.
            New York: Random House.
Imershein, Allen W.
    1977a   "The Epistemological Bases of Social Order:
            Toward Ethnoparadigm Analysis." Chapter 1
            (pp 1-51) in David Heise (ed.), Sociological
            Methodology 1977. Washington: Jossey-Bass.
    1977b   "Organizational Change as a Paradigm Shift."
            Sociological Quarterly 18 (Winter): 33-43.
Lalonde, Marc
    1974   A New Perspective on the Health of Canadians.
            Ottowa: Canadian Ministry of National Health
            and Welfare.
Levin, Lowell S., Alfred H. Katz and Erik Holst
    1976   Self-Care: Lay Initiatives in Health. New
            York; Prodist.
Maxmen, Jerrold S.
    1976   The Post-Physician Era. New York: John Wiley
            and Sons
Mechanic, David
    1976   The Growth of Bureaucratic Medicine. New
            York: John Wiley and Sons.
Metsch, Jonathan M. and James E. Veney
    1976   "Consumer Participation and Social
            Accountability." Medical Care 14 (April):
            282-293.
Milio, Nancy
    1974   "Dimensions of Consumer Participation and
            National Health Legislation." American
            Journal of Public Health 64 (April): 357-363.
Morse, Edward V.
    1979   "The Future Development of Preventive
            Medicine." Unpublished manuscript. Tulane
            University, New Orleans, Louisiana.

Navarro, Vicente
 1973   "National Health Insurance and the Strategy for Change." Health and Society 51 (Spring): 223-251.
 1976   The Political and Economic Determinants of Health Care in Rural America." Inquiry 8 (June): 111-121.
Reeder, Leo G.
 1972   "The Patient-Client as Consumer: Some Observations on the Changing Professional-Client Relationship." Journal of Health and Social Behavior 13 (December): 406-412.
Samuels, Mike and Hal Bennett
 1973   The Well Body Book. New York: Random House.
Sidel, Victor W. and Ruth Sidel
 1976   "Beyond Coping." Social Policy 7: 67-69.
Starr, Paul
 1976   "The Politics of Therapeutic Nihilism." Hastings Center Report (October): 24-30.
 1978   "Medicine and the Waning of Professional Sovereignty." Daedalus 107 (Winter): 175-194.
Stoller, Eleanor Palo
 1974   "New Roles for Health Consumers: A Study in Role Transformation." Paper presented to the American Sociological Association. August.
Stratmann, William, et al
 1975   "A Study of Consumer Attitudes about Health Care: The Control, Cost, and Financing of Health Services." Medical Care 13 (Aug): 659-668.
Task Force on Preventive Medicine
 1976   Preventive Medicine USA. New York: Prodist.
Warren, Roland L., Stephen M. Rose and Ann F. Bergunder
 1974   The Structure of Urban Reform. Lexington: D.C. Heath and Company.
Young, Kue
 1975   "Lay-Professional Conflict in a Canadian Community Health Center: A Case Report." Medical Care 13 (November): 899-904.